THRIVING WITH ADHD

A Guide to Naturally Reducing ADHD Symptoms in Your Child

THRIVING WITH ADHD

A Guide to Naturally Reducing ADHD Symptoms in Your Child

DANA KAY

Copyright © 2022 by Dana Kay

All rights reserved. No part of this book may be used or reproduced in any manner whatsoever without prior written consent of the authors, except as provided by the United States of America copyright law.

Published by Best Seller Publishing®, St. Augustine, FL
Best Seller Publishing® is a registered trademark.
Printed in the United States of America.
ISBN: 978-1-956649-61-1

This publication is designed to provide accurate and authoritative information with regard to the subject matter covered. It is sold with the understanding that the publisher is not engaged in rendering legal, accounting, or other professional advice. If legal advice or other expert assistance is required, the services of a competent professional should be sought. The opinions expressed by the authors in this book are not endorsed by Best Seller Publishing® and are the sole responsibility of the author rendering the opinion.

For more information, please write:
Best Seller Publishing®
53 Marine Street
St. Augustine, FL 32084
or call 1 (626) 765 9750
Visit us online at: www.BestSellerPublishing.org

ADHD Thrive Institute
6947 Coal Creek Pkway SE, PMB #144
Newcastle, WA 98059
book@adhdthriveinstitute.com

Category: Health and Wellness

TO MY DEAR SON, OLIVER.

At the present time, you probably don't comprehend how much you inspired me and drove me to find answers.

At the present time, you probably don't comprehend that you alone changed the trajectory of our family life and my professional career.

At the present time, you probably don't realize that our story—your story—will help thousands of other kids and families out there find peace and happiness.

One day you will comprehend all of this, and when that day comes …

I will truly thank you,
acknowledge you,
and share that I am forever grateful.

I love you (and of course like you)
from the bottom of my heart and soul.

Table of Contents

Acknowledgments ... ix

Introduction ... xi

Chapter 1: Why Food First? ... 1

Chapter 2: The ADHD Diet, Part 1 ... 23

Chapter 3: The ADHD Diet, Part 2 ... 45

Chapter 4: Superfoods ... 67

Chapter 5: GMOs and Organic Produce—What Caregivers Need to Know ... 87

Chapter 6: Meal Planning 101 ... 105

Chapter 7: Hidden Sources of Gluten, Dairy, and Soy ... 119

Chapter 8: What About Supplements? ... 133

Chapter 9: But What About …? Common Obstacles and How to Overcome Them, Part 1 ... 153

Chapter 10: But What About …? Common Obstacles and How to Overcome Them, Part 2 ... 175

Chapter 11: When Food Isn't Enough: The Missing Piece, Part 1 ... 195

Chapter 12: When Food Isn't Enough: The Missing Piece, Part 2 ... 213

Conclusion ... 227

Glossary ... 229

   Code Words for Sugar ... 234

   Code Words for Gluten ... 235

   Code Words for Dairy ... 236

Endnotes ... 239

Acknowledgments

First and foremost, I would like to bring your attention to the dedication page of this book. Oliver deserves the biggest acknowledgment of them all. Without him, this book would not even have been a dream. He has embraced all of the changes I mention throughout this book. There have been challenging moments—like friends' birthday parties, Halloween, and the amounts of candy they hand out at school—but he faced each challenging moment and proved that persistence is more powerful than perfection.

To Martine, my partner in crime, who may not be out in front for all to see but is the glue that holds our business together. Side by side but miles apart, sisters are doin' it for themselves.

To my special hubby, Ben, for putting up with the ticking, clicking, and rattling sounds coming from my keyboard late at night in bed, for reading drafts, for giving me advice on how to not sound too polarizing, and for his unwavering support.

As most parents know, it takes a village, and I would not have been able to bring this book to life without my wonderful team who support and drive this amazing vision on a day-to-day basis. A special call-out to Lindsey Bell, who copyedited the book—her talent, skill, warmth, and precision are gifts that I am so grateful for.

Last but not least, I would like to thank all of my family for their love, encouragement, and support. If I listed all of their names, we would be here all day and I would likely forget to note someone, which I don't want to happen! You know who you are, and I love you all very much.

Introduction

My four-year-old son sat beside me in the waiting room. He was playing on my phone at that moment because I honestly just couldn't take any more of his hyperactivity. Just one moment of peace! It was all I wanted.

"Oliver!" The nurse called us back with a kind smile on her face. "You can go into room 2 and have a seat, please."

The doctor took a chair beside me and explained that my son had attention deficit hyperactivity disorder (ADHD). He handed me a prescription, answered our questions (though to be honest, I didn't really even know what to ask at that moment), and sent us on our way.

"Finally!" I told my husband that evening as we climbed into bed. "We're finally going to get some peace and calm."

I felt my body relax that night like it hadn't in a long time. I sank into my pillow and breathed in the knowledge that we were going to get some relief soon. I always knew there was something different about my sweet son, but it wasn't until this diagnosis that I felt understood. Validated. Heard.

A Ticket Off the Emotional Rollercoaster

I drove to the pharmacy the next day and filled that prescription with my head held high. We were going to get some relief. Things were going to be okay. The meltdowns, hyperactivity, constant impulsive behavior, emotional dysregulation, and walking on eggshells would soon be things of the past. For years we had felt like we were on an emotional rollercoaster, a rollercoaster that wouldn't stop and that we couldn't get off. Finally, we'd found a way. That prescription was going to be our ticket off the rollercoaster. At least, that's what I thought.

I couldn't have been more wrong. Not only did many of these symptoms continue, but Oliver also developed new symptoms—side effects from the medication.

"What should we do now?" I asked the doctor at our next follow-up appointment. "Let's add in another medication," he said as he handed me another prescription designed to counteract the side effects of the first.

Shortly after that, we upped the dosage of one of the medicines and then added a third medication. By the time the doctor was suggesting a fourth, I knew this couldn't be right. There had to be another way that didn't involve pounding his little body with strong prescriptions. What I thought would be one pill quickly turned into four, and my gut told me there had to be other options.

The Interventions No One Ever Mentioned

That's when I started doing some research into natural ADHD treatments. What I found blew me away! Before doing this research, I had wholeheartedly believed medication was the right path for ADHD treatment for every child. In my mind, there was NO OTHER treatment that would be as effective. Yet there was a basic intervention hidden in plain sight: diet. I had no idea diet could impact the body, brain, gut, and behavior so much. Even now, I am not necessarily against medication, but my core concern is about jumping straight into strong stimulant medications for young children, especially when other, more natural approaches can work just as well for some.

But the truth is, diet CAN be just as effective as medication in reducing ADHD symptoms. Sometimes it can even be more effective. The science is clear on that. In fact, diet can also be helpful for those with ASD, anxiety, depression, and other similar disorders. We'll get into the science of this more in the pages to come.

What upset me more than anything else, though, was that no one told us any of this. When Oliver was diagnosed with ADHD, the ONLY treatment option we were provided with was medication. Counseling wasn't suggested. Neither was any form of therapy. When I brought up dietary changes with my doctor, he said, "You can try it if you want, but you'll just be wasting your time."

Why wasn't anyone telling us about the effects that food can have on ADHD symptoms? Why was medication the ONLY option our doctor gave us? How did my son's doctor not know about some of the information I was learning online? There was no conversation about the pros and cons of various interventions. In fact, there weren't any other interventions mentioned. Medication—and medication alone—was it.

That's not okay.

There are other caregivers just like me who are seeing negative side effects from ADHD medications. There are others who would prefer to try natural solutions first. But if doctors aren't even telling them about these solutions, if doctors aren't even aware of these solutions, how are caregivers supposed to know they exist?

Medication Is NOT the Only Way

That's why I wanted to write this book. So that caregivers realize there are other options. ADHD is the most common mental disorder among children in the U.S. today.[1] In 2011, it was estimated that 11 percent of children were diagnosed with ADHD. Back then, that equaled 6.4 million children in the U.S. alone.[2] Those numbers have continued to rise steadily year after year. That means that today, there are millions of children and their families affected by ADHD.

As the founder and CEO of the ADHD Thrive Institute and a Board Certified Holistic Health and Nutrition Practitioner specializing in ADHD, I talk with these caregivers daily. I hear their frustration when medication doesn't work or when they want to avoid medication but don't feel like they have any other options. I listen to their cries as their children scream and yell in the background on our phone calls. My heart breaks for these people, because I was in their shoes years ago.

I know what it's like to cry myself to sleep every night because my child is out of control.

I know what it's like to scour the internet day after day, searching for something—anything—that might help my child. I know what it's like to say out loud, "I don't like my son," and then feel terribly guilty for voicing it.

I know what it's like to find a treatment that other people promise will make all the difference—only to try it on my son and be disappointed. Again.

I'm an ADHD health practitioner, yes, but I'm also a mom of a child with ADHD, and I know how hard this journey is. I've walked it myself, and it is a true honor to be walking it again with you through this book.

Please remember as you read this book, though, that it's not intended as a substitute for the medical advice of physicians. You should always consult a physician in matters relating to health and particularly with respect to symptoms that may require diagnosis or medical attention.

A Road Map

In the pages ahead, I'm going to provide a road map for you that will show you exactly how to use food to naturally reduce ADHD symptoms. In Chapter 1, we'll explore the backbone of natural ADHD symptom reduction: why it works and what the science and real-life experience have taught me. In Chapters 2 and 3, you'll learn what foods to eat for ADHD, as well as what foods to avoid and why. In Chapters 4 and 5, I'll clear up any confusion you might have about superfoods, genetically modified organisms, and organic produce.

In Chapter 6, I'll provide a step-by-step guide to meal planning to remove all the stress and confusion of this often-dreaded task. In Chapter 7, I'll help you avoid a trap that many caregivers I work with fall into. These caregivers think their children are completely gluten-free, only to realize shortly thereafter that there are hidden sources of gluten lurking in their pantry and keeping them from seeing the progress they want to see.

You can't talk about natural ADHD interventions without mentioning supplements! That's what we'll learn about in Chapter 8. In Chapters 9 and 10, I'll explore some of the most common obstacles caregivers of children with ADHD run into when they begin changing their diet. We'll investigate picky eating, financial barriers, difficult family members or friends, and a host of other obstacles caregivers face when beginning this journey.

Finally, in Chapters 11 and 12, we'll look at what to do when a caregiver makes all of these changes and their child is still struggling. It would be nice if we could do one thing that was guaranteed to work. *Just change the food you eat, and your child will no longer struggle.* I wish I could make that promise.

Unfortunately, that's not reality because every child is different, every family is different, and every circumstance is unique. Our children with ADHD are whole people, so sometimes just changing the food they eat isn't enough. Sometimes, we need to dig a little deeper for underlying stressors in their unique bodies. Or, sometimes, we need to look at how we interact as a family. Is it possible that family members have developed new ways of interacting with one another that aren't exactly healthy? We will look at these issues—and more—in Chapters 11 and 12.

There Is Hope

Through it all, I want this book to offer you hope. Hope that there are options for your family. Hope that this isn't the best it's ever going to be. Hope that there are great things ahead for you, for your family, and for your child with ADHD.

Interspersed throughout the pages of this book are stories from families just like yours. Names and details about their stories have been slightly modified, of course, to protect their privacy, but other than these small details, their stories are true. These families have children with ADHD and have been able to successfully navigate the dietary changes I suggest in this book. They've seen just how effective natural solutions can be at reducing ADHD symptoms. I hope their stories encourage you.

Also interspersed throughout the book are QR codes that you can scan to download additional resources. If you're not able to scan the QR codes, we have also included a link to all of the resources in the conclusion of this book. We hope this bonus material is helpful as you take this journey with your family!

Natural solutions work,[3] and I believe with all my heart that you didn't pick up this book by accident. Maybe you picked it up because you want to try a natural solution for your child before you try medication. Maybe you picked it up because you've already tried medicine, and it hasn't gone well. Whatever led you to this book wasn't an accident. You're here because you need help, and my hope is that this book gives you exactly what you need. When I went through this journey with my son years ago, I did it alone. I don't want anyone else to have to do that. When the going gets tough, remember you're not alone in this. I've got you, and you've got this!

CHAPTER 1:
Why Food First?

"Can you *please* sit down?" I gritted my teeth and tried to appear calm and patient as I asked my son again to sit in his chair at our favorite Mexican restaurant. To his credit, he plopped back down when I asked, but it wasn't five minutes later before he was up again. This same charade played over probably fifteen times in our short dinner. Each time I asked him to sit, my frustration and embarrassment grew.

My friend's child, who was sitting right beside my son, didn't get up once during our dinner together. I know because I watched him like a hungry predator watching her next meal all night long. How could he be so calm when my child was so hyper ALL THE TIME? My friend's child colored on his coloring page, not making so much as a peep. They were the same age, my son and my friend's son, but my son was a terror compared to him.

> *What was I doing wrong?*
>
> *Why was my child the only one who seemed to be out of control all the time?*
>
> *Why did nothing ever work?*

Deep in my gut, I always knew there was something a little bit different about my oldest son, Oliver. From a very early age, he seemed to have higher energy levels than other boys. I told myself it was nothing and tried to believe the comments of well-meaning onlookers who said things like, "Boys will be boys," or "All little boys are that active." But all along, my gut told me there was more going on with my son.

As he got older, I started noticing other red flags, flags like:

- An inability to control or calm his mind and body
- Constant struggles to keep his hands to himself
- Lots of fidgeting
- Excessive talking and an inability to wait his turn
- An inability to stay seated
- HUGE meltdowns over the smallest things

These meltdowns sometimes lasted for hours, and they became so prevalent that there were times when I was afraid to leave the house with him, not knowing what he might do in public. The rest of the family was walking on eggshells all the time too, just waiting for the next inevitable tantrum to drop.

His behavior got especially challenging when our second child was born. My body ached with exhaustion from caring for a newborn, and Oliver's energy levels went through the roof. The frequency and intensity of his tantrums increased dramatically. My whole life felt like it was spinning out of control. Each morning, I dragged myself out of bed, dreading what mood my son would be in that day. Each night, I cried myself to sleep, feeling guilty about the negative feelings I had toward my son. I resented him for what he was putting me and our family through but also hated myself for feeling that way.

Overwhelm, exhaustion, and unhappiness were my daily companions.

I watched other parents with their seemingly perfect children and wondered what I was doing wrong. I wanted that picture-perfect family I always imagined us having, but that kind of family life felt far out of reach.

I can still vividly remember the day that opened my eyes to just how far we really were from that picture-perfect family. Oliver and I were in the grocery store, and he wanted to open a snack we hadn't paid for yet. When I said no, he threw a tantrum like I had never seen before. He threw himself on the floor and kicked his legs as he rolled around.

"Stop it. Get up," I said, louder than I should have. He ignored me. By the time I noticed the pasta sauce display near him, it was too late. He flailed his body and kicked one last time, hitting the corner of the display with his foot. Two glass jars shattered beside him, and red sauce went flying.

My face burned with embarrassment. People walked by. Some shook their heads in judgment. Others averted their eyes in an attempt to make me less uncomfortable. I even overheard one mom say under her breath, "Seriously, learn to control your child."

What kind of mom was I? Not only could I not control my son's behavior, but I also couldn't control my own reactions to him.

I broke down right there in the middle of the store—humiliated, defeated, and convinced I was an utter failure as a mom. That was my turning point. I knew we couldn't keep going on like this. Something had to give.

Not long after that, Oliver's teacher started noticing ADHD tendencies too. She suggested we schedule an evaluation with a pediatric psychiatrist.

Upon evaluation, Oliver was diagnosed with ADHD. I took a deep breath, relieved to know there was something to explain his behavior. Finally, I had outside validation that I wasn't making it all up. There really was something, a diagnosable condition that explained his difficult behaviors. More than that, there were medications that would reduce his ADHD symptoms. Now that we knew what we were dealing with, we could finally get some help.

His pediatrician sat us down, explained the diagnosis, and handed us a prescription. For a while, we basked in the benefits of this medication. I remember thinking to myself, "We're finally going to find some peace and calm in our house!"

But then, the bottom fell out. As we increased the dose per the doctor's instructions, Oliver experienced side effects. He became quieter and more withdrawn. He didn't want to eat during the day and couldn't sleep at night. He was anxious all the time. Every afternoon at around 3 pm, he had a huge meltdown—a meltdown that was worse than any he had before we started him on medication. It was as if the medication had worn off, releasing all of his pent-up energy like a volcanic eruption. He wasn't himself.

I called the doctor, and he suggested adding another medication to counteract those side effects. With that medication came other side effects, though, so he suggested another. By the time he was suggesting a fourth medication for my young son, I knew something had to change. We couldn't keep pounding his tiny body with more and more medications.

When Oliver was first diagnosed with ADHD and prescribed medication, I thought that was it. I assumed one medication would give us the results we wanted, and we would be done. Unfortunately, for my family—and for many families I have worked with since then—medication is not a quick fix. We sometimes assume it will be, but that rarely happens.

It can take months—sometimes even years—to find the right medication and dosage. Caregivers have to navigate side effects and track behaviors to see which medication is working and which one isn't. They have to schedule doctors' appointments on a regular basis to discuss their findings and evaluate symptoms. As children grow, dosages change. Sometimes, medications that once worked effectively stop working.

I thought medication would be a quick fix; it was instead a long and arduous journey that ended with Oliver's doctor requesting yet another medication. My son's doctor didn't offer us any other solutions. It was medication or misery.

Unfortunately, since that time, in my work with nearly one thousand families of children with ADHD, I've learned that my experience is far from abnormal. When a child receives an ADHD diagnosis, the first thing doctors typically give caregivers is a prescription. They don't often tell them about the effects of diet on ADHD symptoms. Many of them don't even *know* about the effects of diet on ADHD symptoms. One mom told me that her doctor discouraged her from trying a natural course by saying this: "Sure, you can adjust your child's diet and it might help a little bit, but the *best* course of action is medication."

Who doesn't want the *best* for their child? We all do, of course. When a doctor tells us what the "best" course of treatment is, we trust them because we assume they are the experts. That's exactly what I did for a long time, and it's what many of the families I work with have done too.

Sadly, in trusting the experts, many of us have shoved aside our gut instincts—our instincts that tell us maybe there is another way.

What if, instead of medication, doctors prescribed other things first? Things like dietary or lifestyle changes. Is it possible that dietary changes alone can reduce ADHD symptoms so much that medication is no longer needed or that a lower dosage might be effective? I believe that it is. I am not against medication and definitely think there are instances where it is the BEST course of action, but it concerns me how quickly we jump straight into strong stimulant medications for young children.

That's what we're going to investigate in this book—whether there are other viable options.

But let me go ahead and let you in on a little secret: there are. In my work as a Board Certified Holistic Health and Nutrition Practitioner, specializing in children with ADHD, I have watched families find freedom from ADHD symptoms naturally time and time again. I've also seen it in my own son.

More than that, though, I've read the articles and scientific studies that support natural ADHD symptom reduction. In the next few pages, we're going to look at some of the science. But I do want to be upfront with you right from the beginning. What I'm going to share in this book is not traditionally recognized by the entire medical community. Not all doctors agree that diet can make a significant difference in ADHD symptoms. Some of them feel the findings are inconclusive. Nonetheless, I believe it is more than compelling and that it's 100 percent worth the effort. I have seen success in the natural approach, not only in my own son but also in close to one thousand other children.

The next few pages might get a little academic, but stick with me because I promise it'll be worth it. There is one study in particular that completely changed my life. Are you ready to dive in?

> IF ANY OF THE WORDS MENTIONED IN THE PAGES AHEAD ARE HARD TO KEEP STRAIGHT, FLIP TO THE BACK OF THE BOOK. WE'VE INCLUDED A GLOSSARY OF SOME OF THE KEY TERMS IN THIS BOOK AND THINK IT'LL BE HELPFUL IN THIS RESPECT.

The Gut-Brain Connection

Before we dig into the specific studies that show just how effective dietary modifications can be with ADHD, I want to explain the gut-brain connection. What the gut-brain connection means is that, in essence, our brains are deeply connected to our guts. If our guts aren't functioning well, our brains won't be able to function well either.

Many people don't realize that just about all disease begins in the gut or the digestive system. Eighty percent of the body's entire immune system is within the gut wall, along with billions of nerve cells and an extensive amount of beneficial gut microorganisms (also known as gut bacteria); 90–95 percent of the body's serotonin and 50 percent of the body's dopamine is produced in the gut. These neurotransmitters are the ones that help us manage emotions and balance mood. Do your children with ADHD struggle to manage their emotions? Do they seem to have HUGE mood swings? Then it's likely their bodies—and, in particular, their guts—are not making enough of these vital neurotransmitters.

Emotional dysregulation is a common symptom of ADHD, but many caregivers don't realize that this emotional dysregulation actually starts in the gut, where serotonin and dopamine are made. The problem, then, is not the emotions themselves, but the fact that the correct amounts of these vital neurotransmitters are not being made in the first place. By working to improve gut health, many caregivers of children with ADHD find that the emotional dysregulation problems solve themselves.

The brain has many areas that are involved in gut function, but one of the main areas is the frontal lobe. The frontal lobe talks to the gut via nerve branches and two-way chemical messengers. The frontal lobe is involved in the following:

- Attention
- Focus
- Executive function
- Planning
- Organizing
- Problem-solving

Do any of these areas sound like ones that are affected by ADHD? If you're familiar with common ADHD symptoms, they should! Children with ADHD often struggle with ALL of these tasks. Because the frontal lobe is in the brain, many people are under the impression that the brain is what needs care, when in reality it's also the gut that's causing the problems.

A person's gut health is quite literally connected to everything that occurs in the body. If we are able to improve gut function, then we are able to target not just symptoms but underlying stressors as well.

Think of it this way: have you ever felt butterflies in your stomach because you were nervous about something? Maybe it was a test or a conflict or a first date. These are perfect examples of the gut-brain connection. Our bodies perceive whatever we are nervous about as a stressful situation, and then our brains trigger raw emotions in the gut, resulting in nausea or that feeling of butterflies in the stomach. That's the brain talking to the gut.

But the reverse is also true. Our guts talk to our brains as well. When the digestive system, specifically the intestinal tract, has a higher level of bad gut bacteria than good, it's called gut dysbiosis. Gut dysbiosis creates inflammation that travels through the vagus nerve to the brain. Once this reaches the brain, it creates symptoms like brain fog, confusion, dizziness, poor memory, and a whole host of neuro-behavioral disorders like ADHD, anxiety, and depression.

It's kind of like a highway. The gut and brain are constantly sending messages back and forth. When medication is prescribed for ADHD, it's often to treat the symptoms in the brain alone. But that medication does absolutely nothing about whatever might be going on in the gut.

Think about selective serotonin reuptake inhibitors (SSRIs), for example. These medications are often prescribed to people with depression and anxiety. Serotonin is one of the neurotransmitters that enables brain cells to communicate with one another. It helps with mood stabilization and makes people feel happy. SSRIs make more serotonin accessible in the brain by blocking its reabsorption. In essence, what SSRIs do is help the patient's body better manage the serotonin it currently has. They DON'T actually create more serotonin in the body.

What I'm advocating in this book is that there is a better approach. Instead of treating the symptom (i.e., the fact that serotonin isn't being managed correctly), figure out why the body isn't producing enough serotonin in the first place. Then fix this issue, so the body begins to produce the right amount of serotonin on its own.

It's like a fire. When a house fire breaks out and the emergency responders arrive on the scene, they don't aim their hoses at the smoke. They aim them at the fire. They know that if they get the fire out, the smoke will eventually dissipate. It's the same way with our health. If we aim for the fire (in our case, the underlying stressor), the smoke (or symptoms) will eventually dissipate. But if all we do is flood the smoke with water, we're never actually even touching the problem below. Let's stop shooting water at smoke and start getting to the underlying issues!

Focus on the underlying stressor, not just the symptom on the surface. To focus on the brain and not the gut is counterproductive. It doesn't make sense because the brain and the gut are connected to each other and they're constantly communicating.

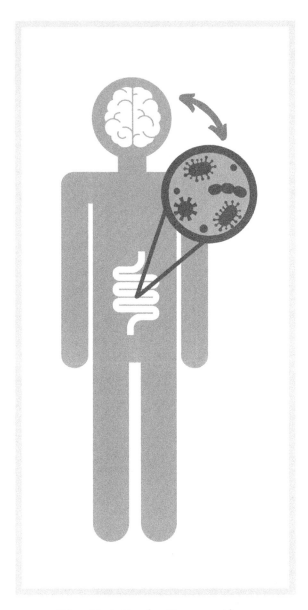

The Gut-Brain Connection

The digestive system (aka the gut) is responsible for receiving food, breaking it down, extracting the nutrients, and discarding the junk. If at any point in doing these things the digestive system is impaired, it wreaks havoc on the entire body. One of the primary ways I see this in my practice is with a leaky gut. Leaky gut can be caused by parasites, toxic exposure, medication, gluten, food intolerances, or other underlying stressors.

Leaky gut is when food particles slip through the intestinal walls and head into the bloodstream. When this occurs, the body recognizes these food particles as foreign matter and then creates an immunological response.[4]

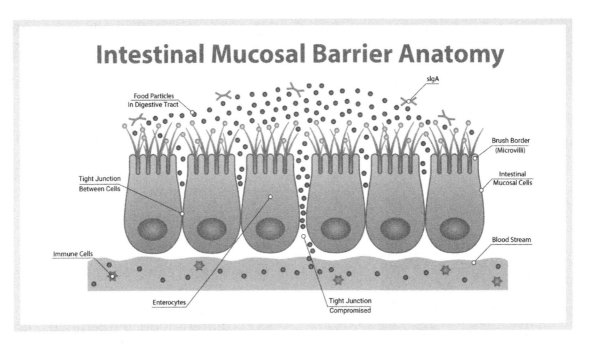

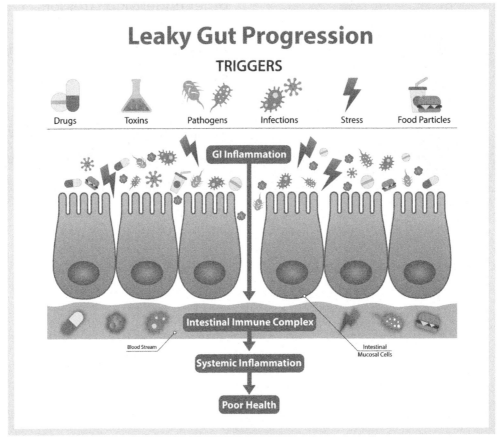

Leaky gut might show up in the following ways:

- Inflammation in the body
- Malabsorption of essential nutrients
- Transfer of toxins to the brain (resulting in poor concentration, poor memory, anxiety, depression, or behavioral issues)
- Anxiety or depression
- Constipation or diarrhea
- ADHD symptoms
- Emotional dysregulation
- Autoimmune disorders
- Skin conditions such as rashes or eczema
- Frequent colds or flu
- Food sensitivities, intolerance, or allergies

If the gut isn't functioning properly, many other areas of the body are affected. It's not only the stomach.

When Sarah came to me, her son didn't have any issues that were obviously gut-related. He went to the bathroom daily and didn't have hard stools or diarrhea. He didn't have stomachaches either. His only symptom that Sarah mentioned was emotional dysregulation.

"When he doesn't get what he wants," she told me, "he just completely loses it! He screams and kicks and just completely flips out."

I asked Sarah what foods he ate. "Typical kid food," she told me, "like hot dogs, chicken nuggets, and pizza." I worked with Sarah to change her son's diet, and then we did functional lab tests for them.

We'll get into functional lab testing more in a later chapter, but if you'd like to get a sneak peek, I invite you to check out a video training session I did on leaky gut and functional lab testing.

TO WATCH THIS VIDEO, SCAN THE FOLLOWING QR CODE:

The functional lab tests showed us that Sarah's son did, in fact, have a leaky gut. Even though he had no "gut symptoms," his body was still suffering because of poor gut health. Once she worked to improve his leaky gut, his emotional dysregulation completely disappeared. Sarah told me just the other day, "He's like a different kid now. He's happy."

Sometimes the symptoms our children display don't seem connected to the gut, but most of the time they are. The gut is connected to everything.

Thankfully, leaky gut isn't a death sentence. It's not permanent. It can be corrected, and it can be done without medication through dietary modifications. We'll dive into that in a later chapter. Now that you understand WHY the gut plays such an important role in ADHD, let's look at what the science says.

The Science Is Far from Silent

As mentioned earlier, it was the science that first made me rethink the direction we were traveling with my son, Oliver—that and the fact that he was having significant side effects from medication. It was the science that convinced me natural methods were worth a shot. It's important to understand, though, that not all medical professionals agree with the natural approach. Some doctors believe the evidence is inconclusive.

I'm going to let you decide, because the truth is, you have to do what's best for your family. Follow your gut. Trust your instincts. We tried the medication route and saw significant negative side effects. Then we tried the natural route and saw significant improvement. I've also seen significant improvement in close to one thousand other families, so I believe the natural method is worth a shot. Keep reading, and then trust your instincts because you know your child better than anyone else.

A study in 2011[5] concluded that 64 percent of children diagnosed with ADHD were actually experiencing a hypersensitivity to food. Did you catch that? Sixty-four percent! I wonder what might happen if these children changed their diets and removed the foods they were sensitive to. Is it possible these ADHD symptoms would disappear or at least become more manageable? I believe it is.

Another study showed that 56 percent of ADHD kids tested positive for food allergies compared to less than 8 percent of kids in the general population.[6] That tells me there is a clear correlation between ADHD and food allergies. Nonetheless, most doctors don't even mention this correlation to caregivers.

In 2002, a study[7] was done to show the connection between food intolerances and depression. The study concluded that the patients' symptoms of depression considerably improved while on an elimination diet. Granted, this study was about depression, not ADHD, but considering what we know about the neurotransmitters that are made in the gut (serotonin and dopamine), it makes sense that if a similar study were conducted on patients with ADHD, there would likely be similar results.

In 2015, a study[8] showed the risk of hyperactivity increased by 14 percent with each additional sweetened beverage. It also correlated soda consumption with higher aggression. And yet, even though these are two common symptoms of ADHD in children, caregivers are rarely told to avoid soda.

In 2017, a study[9] concluded that the addition of micronutrients in the diet improved overall function, reduced impairments, and improved attention, emotional regulation, and aggression. Clearly, medication is NOT the only way to help children with ADHD.

All of these studies strongly suggest that diet matters, but the study that really blew me away was conducted by the Autism Research Institute.[10] In this study, the researchers compared the behavioral effects of different types of interventions to see which ones were most effective. To do this, they looked at data they had been collecting from parents since 1967. They reviewed interventions such as amphetamine medication, antibiotics, antifungals, sleeping medicines, SSRIs, certain vitamins and supplements, and various special diets.

The researchers collated the responses and combined them into three categories: symptoms were made worse, treatment had no effect, or symptoms were made better. The "Better to Worse" column gives the number of children who "Got Better" compared to each child who "Got Worse." This ratio is the one that finally convinced me of just how effective dietary changes are in reducing ADHD symptoms. See the chart that follows.

With many of the common ADHD medications, for every child who got better, another got worse. Can you believe that? Is this disturbing to anyone else? Why are doctors prescribing medication as the first plan of treatment if the medications only help about half of the children prescribed them and if the other half actually get worse?

I'm here to tell you there is a better way. You don't have to settle for a 50 percent chance that your child might get better and a 50 percent chance that they'll get worse.

Parent Ratings

Special Diets	Got Worse	No Effect	Got Better	Better: Worse	No. of Cases
Gluten/Casein-Free Diet	3%	28%	69%	24:1	3593
Removed Milk Products/Dairy	2%	44%	55%	32:1	6950
Removed Sugar	2%	46%	52%	27:1	4589
Removed Wheat	2%	43%	55%	30:1	4340

Look at the special diets section of the previous chart. Parents who implemented a gluten-free and casein-free diet for their children showed a 24:1 ratio. That means that for every twenty-four kids who got better, only one child got worse. Now look at the sugar column. Parents who removed sugar saw a 27:1 ratio, meaning that twenty-seven children improved, while only one child worsened. (And, most likely, the one child who did worsen was probably going through sugar withdrawal!)

The difference in the effectiveness between medications and dietary intervention is huge, and this study clearly indicates that changing a child's diet will be more effective for most families than popping a pill. (If you'd like to see the full research article, check it out in the references listed at the back of this book.)

So why isn't dietary intervention THE go-to intervention? Your guess is as good as mine, but this needs to change. Dietary interventions are not only MORE effective in many families, according to this study, but they are also side-effect free. Caregivers who are changing their child's diet don't have to worry about dangerous side effects that are often associated with strong medications. Really, there's nothing to lose with the natural approach.

Katie's Story

Katie's daughter had ADHD, as well as oppositional defiant disorder (ODD), when I met her. Katie had taken her to specialist after specialist, grasping at anything that might make their life less challenging. What did each of these specialists suggest?

You got it. More medication. Every single specialist she saw suggested another prescription. Not one of them said anything to Katie about the effectiveness of dietary changes on behavior.

Unfortunately, none of the medications they suggested created positive changes in her daughter. Some of them actually made things worse. Katie told me about one time when they went to a family dinner at her parents' house. Katie had just introduced a new ADHD medication, hoping that maybe this one would be the right fit. Sadly, it wasn't.

"I want another one!" Her daughter grabbed for the plate of chocolate chip cookies that sat on the kitchen counter.

"I'm sorry, sweetie, but three cookies is enough," Katie told her. She braced herself for what she knew was going to happen next—the inevitable tantrum that would follow her refusal to give her daughter exactly what she had asked for.

"That's not fair!" she screamed. "I never get what I want!"

Katie grabbed for the plate to move it to another location where it wouldn't be in her daughter's line of sight, but just as she did that Katie's daughter grabbed her arm.

"NO!" she yelled again. "Give them back! Give them back! I want another one!" She pressed her tiny little fingernails into Katie's arm. It was like she was saying, "If you won't give me what I want willingly, I'll force you to!"

Right then, Katie's parents walked in to see what the noise was all about. Katie's face went red, and she felt the tears of embarrassment pooling behind her eyes.

No, she told herself, *I'm not going to cry right now. Not in front of my parents. Then again, they already see just how much of a failure I am. I can't even keep my daughter from attacking me.*

When Katie shared this story with me, my heart broke with hers. I remember what that was like. I remember how embarrassed I used to be by Oliver's behavior and by my inability to get it under control.

Katie's story is similar to many other stories I have heard from caregivers of children with ADHD. They try medication, hoping for positive results. But instead, their children become more aggressive, sometimes even violent. One mom shared with me that her eight-year-old son, two days after trying a new medication for his ADHD, put a hole in his bedroom door.

It's time for something to change! It's time for the first line of treatment to be FOOD, rather than a prescription that has a 50 percent chance of making things worse! Are you with me?

Chapter Highlights

- Medication or misery is NOT the only option for ADHD. Many caregivers are finding that their children with ADHD can have freedom from symptoms without popping a pill. It is possible!

- There is a HUGE connection between gut health and brain health. It's counterproductive to pop a pill to treat the brain while at the same time ignoring the gut. Work on gut health FIRST, and then the rest of the body will improve as well.

- The science is clear: diet DOES matter! In fact, some studies show that dietary changes are MORE effective than medication at reducing ADHD symptoms.

Action Steps

1. Scan this QR code to gain access to a training video about leaky gut and functional lab testing.

2. Review the chapter highlights. Underline any that speak to you today.

3. What's your ADHD story? Take a few minutes to write out your story on the lines provided. Include the following: when you first knew your child might have ADHD, what struggles you are currently facing, what the doctors have suggested to your family, how you feel about these suggestions, and your motivation for picking up this book.

Your ADHD Story

CHAPTER 2:

The ADHD Diet, Part 1

"I don't buy it."

I appreciated Kevin's honesty. Really, I did. But how could I convince him to give dietary changes a shot when he was so against it? Kevin's wife was fully on board and ready to make the dietary changes I suggested. But Kevin wasn't sold on the approach yet.

I offered him a deal. "Cut gluten 100 percent for three months. I know that'll be hard, but I want you to try it for three months. I'm not telling you to commit for life. Just three months. Then, if you do that and don't see any changes, go back to how you were eating."

They talked it over that evening and called me back the next day. "Okay, we'll give you three months." Kevin still didn't think it would actually do anything to help their family, but to appease his wife, he agreed to try it.

Kevin's not the first one to question the natural approach to ADHD. I questioned it myself initially. Years ago, before I became a Holistic Health and Nutrition Practitioner, I was clueless about health and wellness. I worked in accounting. As I said in Chapter 1, I believed the doctors and professionals who told me the best way to treat ADHD was with medication.

It was the science that convinced me otherwise—in particular that study from the Autism Research Institute, referenced in Chapter 1. I read that article and couldn't believe it! *Food can make that much of a difference in behavior? No way!*

After reading that article, I scoured the internet for more information. What foods, in particular, were the worst? Why these foods? In this chapter, I'm going to share that information with you. I had to complete years of tertiary education to learn this information, but I don't think it should be that difficult for anyone else. You shouldn't have to have a degree to know which foods are the worst for children with ADHD.

In fact, I believe many of the foods available in the United States shouldn't be allowed at all—for anyone. Did you know there are food additives and chemicals allowed into food in the United States that are banned either partially or entirely or require warning labels in other countries?[11]

One of these is brominated vegetable oil, a food additive that originates from bromine, which at the very least can irritate the skin and the mucous membranes, but might also lead to memory loss, loss of muscle coordination, or other complications. This additive is banned by the European Union and several other countries, but the United States continues to allow its use in soda. Some other banned ingredients or ingredients that require warning labels in other countries (which you likely have in your pantry or fridge) include genetically modified fruits and veggies, which we will discuss in a later chapter, potassium bromate, Red 40, Yellow 5, Yellow 6, azodicarbonamide, olestra, and others.

It's baffling to me that the United States continues to allow ingredients into the food supply that are not even food. It's no wonder we have so many staggering health issues. We are feeding our bodies things that aren't meant to be food. Unfortunately, many of these ingredients make their way into the foods we feed our children and negatively impact their ADHD symptoms.

In the pages to come, we're going to look at the top food culprits affecting children with ADHD. Which foods are the worst for them, and why? How might these foods in particular be exacerbating their ADHD symptoms? Stick with me as we dive in.

Culprit #1: Gluten

Gluten is the number one food I recommend ALL children with ADHD cut out of their diets. In fact, gluten is so inflammatory that I suggest everyone (even those without ADHD or a known gluten intolerance) stop eating it. Plain and simple, gluten is harmful for everyone. That's because gluten triggers increased intestinal permeability in EVERYONE,[12] even those who don't show an allergic response to it.

Intestinal permeability refers to the breakdown of the intestinal walls. When functioning properly, the walls of the intestines form a barrier, allowing water and nutrients to pass through but blocking other things from entering the bloodstream. When a person has increased intestinal permeability, that can lead to something called leaky gut. If you remember from Chapter 1, leaky gut[13] basically means the tight junctions in the gut that are supposed to control what passes through the lining of the intestines aren't doing their job effectively. They are allowing toxins and other harmful substances to enter the bloodstream that aren't supposed to be there.

What do you imagine happens when these toxic substances enter the bloodstream? If you're thinking, "The body fights them off and tries to get rid of them," you're correct. When something enters the bloodstream that isn't supposed to be there, it triggers an inflammatory response as the body seeks to rectify the issue.

In summary, gluten leads to increased intestinal permeability, which leads to leaky gut,[14] which leads to inflammation, which leads to additional symptoms like stomachaches, constipation, brain fog, inattention, reflux, hyperactivity, chronic runny noses, anger issues, wheezing, and more. Many of these symptoms sound like ADHD, don't they? That's because they are. By cutting out gluten, caregivers of children with ADHD are removing one food that significantly contributes to inflammation in their body. In my experience, caregivers who remove this food, along with the other foods I suggest in the rest of this chapter, find that ADHD symptoms diminish significantly and sometimes disappear completely.

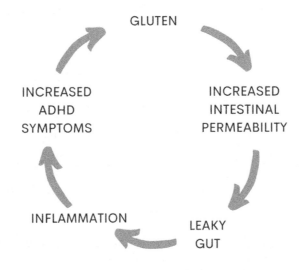

The body doesn't have fences inside it that isolate certain areas. If there is inflammation in one area of the body, that inflammation can spread quickly and easily. Remember the gut-brain connection we learned about in Chapter 1 and how it's like a communication highway between the two? That inflammation that might start in the gut moves quickly to the brain. That's why it makes no sense whatsoever to treat the symptoms without addressing the underlying stressor (in this case, the leaky gut caused by gluten).

Inflammation isn't the only issue with gluten, though. Gluten also has the potential to create opiate-like effects in some individuals. You might want to read that sentence a second time to let it really sink in. Gluten has the potential to act like an OPIATE in the brain. Yes, an OPIATE! Crazy, right?

In individuals who have gut inflammation, which is very common in kids with ADHD, the enzymes in their guts are not fully breaking down gluten. This results in the formation of compounds called gluteomorphins. The protein structure of gluteomorphins is similar to that of morphine. Gluteomorphins are absorbed into the bloodstream, cross the blood-brain barrier, and then bind to opiate receptors in the brain and gastrointestinal tract.

Think about people who are addicted to morphine. They might be unable to sit still. They could have huge meltdowns over small things. They might be unable to handle transitions. In many ways, they have ADHD-like symptoms. When caregivers of children with ADHD remove gluten—and thus remove gluteomorphin—these opiate-like instances begin to be fewer and further in-between.

When we removed gluten from my son's diet, he became a completely different child. Calm. Focused. Able to sit still. Kate said the same thing about her son. In fact, about a month after removing gluten from his diet, she went to dinner with her father-in-law. Typically, her son couldn't sit still for five minutes at the dinner table, let alone for longer stretches of time, making it impossible for Kate to enjoy conversation with family.

"We typically just drove separately to family dinners," she told me. "That way, I could leave as soon as he finished eating, and my husband could enjoy the rest of the mealtime."

They didn't drive separately this time around, though, and Kate feared the worst.

"I just knew we were setting ourselves up for failure. You wouldn't believe it, though. My husband's dad—about halfway through dinner—asked me what medicine we were giving our son." Kate laughed. "He couldn't believe it was food alone that was responsible for Adam's behavior transformation."

Yet, when you think about how opioids affect the body, and when you understand that gluten can create a similar effect, it makes sense that removing gluten can significantly reduce troubling behavior.

Thus far, we have covered two reasons to remove gluten: because it creates inflammation in the body that can exacerbate ADHD symptoms and because it creates an opioid-like addiction. There is one final reason to remove gluten from the diet of a child with ADHD, and that is the glutamate effect.

Glutamate is an amino acid that is both produced in the body and found naturally in many foods. There are also forms of glutamate that do not occur naturally in the body or in food. Have you ever heard of MSG? MSG is monosodium glutamate, and as you have probably guessed, it is made in a lab and doesn't occur naturally. Many people are familiar with the dangers of MSG, but the truth is, an overabundance of naturally occurring glutamate can be damaging as well, especially to children who are already battling inflammation in their bodies.[15]

Some foods that have higher amounts of glutamate in them include tomatoes, cheese, mushrooms, broccoli, walnuts, and wheat. Some of these foods, as you can see, are actually very healthy. The problem arises when there is a buildup of free glutamate in the body. In essence, glutamate that naturally occurs isn't bad unless there's too much of it. One of the best ways to lower the amount of glutamate in the body is to get rid of gluten.

Those three reasons combined are why I suggest families of children with ADHD remove gluten from their diets. Hopefully, I've convinced you to remove it from your diet as well! But maybe you're wondering now what foods contain gluten.

Here are some of the most common sources of gluten:

- All types of bread (except gluten-free, of course): wheat, white, French, sourdough, etc.
- Barley
- Rye
- Pastas (unless specified gluten-free)
- Breading on fried chicken or other fried foods
- Kamut
- Spelt
- Pastries, muffins, pancakes, and waffles (unless specified gluten-free)
- Cookies, cakes, and brownies (unless gluten-free)
- Crackers (unless gluten-free)
- Sauces or gravies if they have been thickened with regular flour

In a later chapter, we'll look at some other hidden sources of gluten, but this gives you a place to start.

One thing to keep in mind when removing gluten is that some people go through a glutamorphin withdrawal response. Think of this like a detox period. During this period, their ADHD symptoms might actually get worse for a time before they get better. That's because their bodies are flushing out the gluten.

Another thing to keep in mind is that it can take three to even six months for gluten to stop reacting in the body. Don't give up if you don't see results immediately! Sometimes, it can take a few months before the body fully reduces the inflammation caused by gluten. Many families ask me if it's okay to eat a little bit of gluten here or there. They assume that a small amount won't hinder their progress. In reality, though, eating small amounts of gluten here or there CAN definitely hinder progress.

Culprit #2: Dairy

Dairy, like gluten, also creates a significant inflammatory response in the body. It is the second most inflammatory food, and about 50 percent of those who have a gluten sensitivity also react to dairy. In fact, some researchers suggest that three out of every four people have an unknown sensitivity to dairy.[16] The main inflammatory protein in dairy is called casein. Casein has a similar protein structure to gluten, and the body reacts in a very similar way.

In fact, the three reasons I suggest families remove gluten are the same reasons I suggest they remove dairy. Dairy products, like gluten, are inflammatory, create opioid-like responses in the brain, and are high in glutamate. The opioid-like protein in dairy is called casomorphin.

Cow's milk naturally contains a cocktail of 35 hormones and growth factors. These are meant for a calf and perfectly suit their growth and development needs. After all, a calf reaches adult size within one year of birth, so it makes sense that they would need a lot of hormones in a very short amount of time. These hormones are perfect for a developing cow, but they aren't designed for human consumption. That's why they can cause damage to the human body.

Dairy intolerance can create digestive problems, allergies, acne, asthma, and a whole host of other issues.

"But what about calcium?" Stacy grew up on a dairy farm, so the thought of removing dairy from her daughter's diet seemed incomprehensible. She had heard all her life that milk was the GO-TO source of calcium. If she cut dairy, wouldn't her daughter's bones become weaker?

"There are actually plenty of other ways to get calcium into the diet," I reassured her. We really don't HAVE to have a glass of milk each day. There are other, better ways to get that calcium into our children's bodies. We'll address this more in a later chapter.

Here are some of the most common sources of dairy:

- Milk
- Cheese
- Yogurt
- Coffee creamers
- Butter
- Ice cream
- Milk chocolate

- Cream cheese
- Sour cream
- Many baked and packaged goods such as muffins, pancakes, cookies, cakes, etc. (unless specified dairy-free)
- Some salad dressings and sauces

> **3 REASONS TO SAY GOODBYE TO GLUTEN AND DAIRY:**
> - THEY BOTH CREATE INFLAMMATION IN THE BODY.
> - THEY BOTH CREATE AN OPIOID-LIKE EFFECT IN THE BRAIN.
> - THEY BOTH LEAD TO EXCESSIVE AMOUNTS OF GLUTAMATE.

Culprit #3: Soy

Soy is the third food children with ADHD should cut from their diets. There are two primary reasons for this. First of all, approximately 95 percent of soy products come from crops of genetically modified organisms (GMOs). GMOs are linked to many health problems. They damage the digestive system and kill off the good bacteria in your gut. We will discuss GMOs in more detail in a later chapter, but suffice it to say they are NOT good for the body and, in particular, for gut health. Because most of the soy in foods today comes from GMO plants, it's best to cut soy out of the diet altogether.

Furthermore, the over-production of soy is a problem in itself. Soy is among the largest United States farm commodities. It's heavily processed, has a high yield, and often contains glyphosate (pesticide) residue. Because of its mass production, it has also sneaked into a variety of foods at an alarming rate.

The second reason I suggest families of children with ADHD remove soy is because soy is an endocrine disruptor. When eaten in excess, it can have adverse effects on the balance of hormones in your body. It also contains isoflavones, which act like estrogen in the body. Since many breast cancers need estrogen to grow, eating an excess of soy could increase the risk of breast cancer.

You might be surprised by how many common products like the ones listed below contain soy:

- Tofu
- Soymilk
- Edamame
- Soy sauce
- Miso
- Baked goods (like breads, cookies, crackers, etc.)
- Canned soups
- Cereals
- Breakfast/energy bars
- Ice cream
- Frozen dinners
- Many dairy-free products like yogurts, milk, cheese, etc.
- Canned meats or lunchmeat
- Vegetable oil

- Chips (check for soybean oil)
- Nut butters (check for soybean oil)
- Worcestershire sauce, as well as other sauces, salad dressings, and gravies

> **2 REASONS TO SAY SEE YA LATER TO SOY:**
> - MOST SOY COMES FROM GENETICALLY MODIFIED ORGANISMS (WHICH ARE LINKED TO MANY HEALTH PROBLEMS).
> - SOY IS AN ENDOCRINE DISRUPTOR AND CAN CAUSE HORMONAL IMBALANCES WITHIN THE BODY.

Culprit #4: Sugar

Gluten, dairy, and soy are the top three inflammatory foods children with ADHD should avoid. Sugar is culprit number four. Many caregivers overlook the importance of blood-sugar management because they think of it in connection with diabetes, not ADHD. In reality, though, blood-sugar management is important for all of us, whether we have diabetes or not.

Unstable blood sugar contributes to a whole host of problems, including an inability to focus and concentrate, increased anxiety and fatigue, an inability to sit still, digestive problems like constipation or diarrhea, a weakened immune system, and so much more. A sudden blood-sugar rise can create hyperactivity or anxiety, whereas a sudden drop in blood sugar can create a sluggish feeling, crankiness, or lack of focus.

Anyone with elevated levels of blood sugar can experience adverse effects on mood and executive functioning, along with a number of additional health issues. Take a look at the following list of symptoms for hypoglycemia (low blood sugar), and think about how similar they are to ADHD symptoms:

- Difficulty listening
- Inability to focus or stay on task
- Being easily distracted
- Quick to get frustrated, and sometimes hard to calm down
- Unexpected anger and lashing out
- Inability to sit still

Do any of these symptoms sound like your child with ADHD? When my son was really struggling, he had every one of these symptoms in excess.

It makes me wonder, are children who are struggling with these behaviors actually battling ADHD symptoms? Or is it fluctuating blood sugar? There's no way to know as long as the child continues to eat excessive amounts of sugar.

One of the moms I have been working with approached me with a problem she was having with her son's school. "The school does great about respecting our requests for all food to be gluten-, dairy-, and soy-free. They don't give him anything without my permission. I'm thankful for that. But today, his teacher asked me for more candy to keep on hand for him. This is the fourth bag I've provided in just a month of school. Apparently, the teachers hand out multiple pieces of candy every day to students as a reward for following instructions. I don't want my son to feel left out, but I'm also concerned about the amount of sugar he is consuming!"

Does this seem counterproductive to anyone else? Why are schools handing out candy (which is scientifically proven to negatively affect behavior) to students who are already struggling? This little guy works so hard to stay calm and focused throughout the day and to keep his hyperactivity in check, but the school is making it even harder!

It's time for the system to change. Food, especially candy, should not be the go-to reward for students.

The ADHD symptoms many children battle can be tied directly to fluctuating blood sugar. One of the best forms of blood-sugar management is the reduction of sugar. Another is eating a low-carbohydrate diet.

There are two main types of carbohydrates: simple and complex. Simple carbs are found in sugary drinks, candy, and other foods that provide little to no nutritional benefit like cookies, crackers, chips, and bakery items. These foods can wreak havoc on children with ADHD. Simple carbohydrates raise blood glucose extremely fast and, as the saying goes, what goes up must come down. The blood sugar spikes rapidly and then falls just as fast, resulting in sluggish, unfocused behavior. Simple carbs should be avoided or seriously limited.

Complex carbs, on the other hand, come from vegetables, whole grains, beans, nuts, and seeds. Complex carbs help sustain steady blood-sugar levels, meaning they do not cause a rapid spike and decline in blood sugar.

One study[17] concluded that the more sugar hyperactive children consume, the more destructive and restless they become. Another study[18] showed a clear correlation between ADHD and children who drink sugar-sweetened beverages. Children with ADHD do NOT need another thing to make them more impulsive, hyperactive, or restless; they battle it enough as it is without sugar heaping on additional challenges.

Researchers have been studying the correlation between sugar and ADHD for quite some time, and this is what one study[19] noted:

- Sugar is a powerful trigger for dopamine release in the brain. (Dopamine is one of the brain chemicals thought to be involved in ADHD). Eating sugar floods brain cells with dopamine, which feels good because dopamine is our pleasure and reward neurotransmitter.

- As people consume sugar, their bodies get used to it being there. The brain then builds up a tolerance to the dopamine and will continue to try to get dopamine production back to normal. This is achieved by reducing the number of dopamine receptors, so it will then take even more sugar to produce the same effect, resulting in a resistance that contributes to even more cravings.

- If a person keeps eating sugar, there may be times when brain cells run low on dopamine from being stimulated so frequently. Low dopamine activity is one of the possible causes of ADHD symptoms. This vicious cycle may also lead to binge eating and sugar addiction.

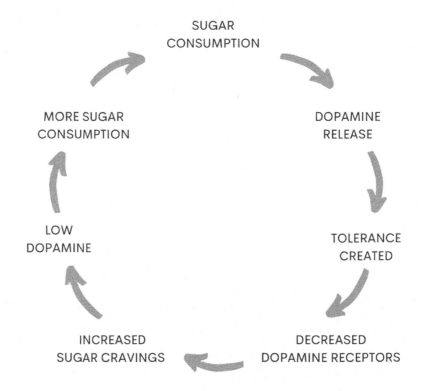

The American Heart Association recommends that children between the ages of two and eighteen should have less than 25 grams (6 teaspoons) of ADDED sugar daily. However, in my experience working with children with ADHD, this amount should be cut in half. Caregivers should aim for less than 12 grams (3 teaspoons) of ADDED sugar daily. This does not include natural sugars found in fruits and vegetables.

What can be tricky is that sugar can be called so many different things. Some code words for sugar include the following:

- Lactose
- Maltose
- Dextrose
- Glucose

- Xylose
- Saccharose
- Sucrose
- Corn sweetener
- Corn syrup
- Corn syrup solids
- Dehydrated cane juice
- Dextrin
- Maltodextrin
- Malt syrup
- Molasses
- Rice syrup
- Sorghum or sorghum syrup

Did you notice that many of these sugars end in -ose? When looking at ingredient labels, look for these -ose words and avoid them as much as possible. The less sugar you and your family eat, the healthier you will be.

Culprit #5: Artificial Flavors and Colors

The final culprits caregivers can remove from their child's diet to help reduce ADHD symptoms are artificial flavors and colors. In the beginning of this chapter, I told you about the sad reality that the United States allows certain chemicals into the food supply that other countries ban, restrict, or require a warning label for. Artificial flavors and colors are some of these restricted items.

ADDitude magazine released an updated article about the effects of artificial flavors and colors on ADHD and said this:

> Studies published in *The Lancet, Pediatrics*, and the *Journal of Pediatrics* suggest that food additives adversely affect a population of children with ADHD ... Two studies from the United Kingdom are good examples. In 2004, one studied healthy preschoolers after giving them either a placebo or 20 milligrams of artificial dye mix plus sodium benzoate. They found that, when the children received the actual dye and sodium benzoate, they had a significant increase in hyperactivity. In the second, in 2007, a research team led by UK researcher Donna McCann studied a group of 3-year-olds and 8- or 9-year-olds. It found that both hyperactive children and non-hyperactive children experienced increased hyperactivity scores when given artificial food colors and additives, suggesting that the dyes are a general public health concern. Starting in 2010, the European Union required the following warning label for all food that contains artificial dye: "May have adverse effect on activity and attention in children."[20]

Even though the Center for Science and the Public Interest has asked the Food and Drug Administration (FDA) to add a warning to these products in the U.S., the FDA refused to do so. They claimed—despite the evidence—that these artificial flavors and colors are safe.

What I think it boils down to is this: The European Union added the warning label to their foods because it chose to restrict the usage of artificial colors until they are proven SAFE. The United States, in contrast, has chosen to continue their usage until they are proven DANGEROUS.

That leaves caregivers today with two options. Like the European Union, they can avoid artificial colors until they know they are actually safe (which will probably never happen) OR, like the United States, they can continue to allow artificial colors into their family's foods and hope they aren't hurting them in the long run. I have chosen to side with the European Union, and I hope you will too! Wouldn't you rather err on the side of caution? Wouldn't you rather avoid items that might be (probably are) dangerous, even if some people aren't fully convinced?

Consumers can eat the same type of food in Britain and the United States and eat very different ingredients. In Britain, they would eat foods made with real ingredients. Actual food! But in the United States, they would eat chemicals disguised as food. Companies use different formulas for U.S. consumers than for those outside the United States. This needs to change! Consumers in the U.S. should be offered the same ingredients as those outside the United States, rather than their chemical counterparts.

Thankfully, things are beginning to change, but not fast enough in my opinion. Several companies have made changes in their product lines to get rid of artificial colors. Unfortunately, there are still MANY companies that refuse to remove artificial flavors and colors from their formulas. You and I can help make this happen by changing the way we eat.

Companies might not listen to our voices, but they will listen to our money. If enough of us refuse to buy products that contain artificial food coloring, they will be forced to make a change.

Will you join me in this task? If so, scan this QR code to gain access to a printable list of ingredients to avoid. Take this list with you anytime you shop. As you look at ingredient lists on labels, avoid all of the products on this list.

The Rest of Kevin's Story

"I'm so glad my wife convinced me to give this a shot."

Kevin's email came at the end of a long week. Being a voice for natural ADHD solutions and speaking out about things that need to change in our food supply can be draining at times. On that particular day, I was spent. Discouraged. Beaten down.

Kevin's words, though, reminded me why I do what I do.

He went on, "You wouldn't believe the changes we have seen in our son. He's like a different kid."

I could believe the changes, though, because I see them all the time. When we remove the inflammatory foods, the body begins to mend itself. And when the body begins to mend, it can function at its best. It can allow our children to become the people we always knew they could be.

Chapter Highlights

- Three reasons to say goodbye to gluten and dairy:
  - They create inflammation in the body
  - They create an opioid-like effect in the brain
  - They can lead to excessive amounts of glutamate
- Two reasons to say see ya later to soy:
  - Most soy comes from genetically modified organisms (which are linked to many health problems)
  - Soy is an endocrine disruptor and can cause hormonal imbalances within the body
- Sugar, when found naturally in whole fruit and vegetables, is a healthy part of a balanced eating plan. Added sugar, usually found in processed foods, sweet drinks, and treats, should be kept to a minimum or eliminated.
- Artificial food coloring can wreak havoc on ALL children, but especially those with ADHD. Avoid it!
- Top five foods children with ADHD should avoid:
  - Gluten
  - Dairy
  - Soy
  - Excessive sugar
  - Artificial flavors and colors

Action Steps

1. Scan this QR code to download a list of ingredients to avoid. Take this list with you anytime you shop. As you look at labels, avoid all of the products on this list.

2. Go through your pantry and pull out all items that contain gluten, dairy, soy, artificial flavors and colors, or excessive amounts of sugar. You don't need to toss them all, but by pulling them out, you get an idea of what products you need to find alternatives to once they are gone. (We'll get into this more in the next chapter.)

CHAPTER 3:

The ADHD Diet, Part 2

I tossed the loaf of bread in the trash bin. Then I grabbed the crackers and packaged cookies. Then the cake mixes. Then the boxes of cereal and cereal bars. I can only imagine what I looked like—some crazed woman ransacking her own home. I threw them all into the trash can until it was too full to close. Shoving it all down with my foot, I made room for more and moved on to the fridge.

I opened the milk, poured it down the sink, and shoved the empty jug into the overflowing trash can. Then I added cheese, yogurt, and sour cream. It was right about then that my husband walked in.

"What in the world are you doing?" He was holding his tongue. I knew he wanted to say more. His eyes *were* definitely saying more.

While there's no right or wrong way to make the dietary changes I suggested in the last chapter, I definitely don't recommend doing it the way I did. Tossing everything out cold turkey was NOT the best approach to healthier living.

Going cold turkey might sound good in theory. After all, the quicker you remove the inflammatory foods, the quicker you'll see results, right? What I didn't take into account, though, was that I had no idea what foods would replace the ones I had tossed. I also didn't think through the amount of pushback I might face from my two young children and husband by making all of these changes so quickly—not to mention that I literally threw away hundreds of dollars' worth of food when I ransacked our kitchen.

Two weeks after my rampage, I plopped down on my bedroom floor, rolled into a ball with my knees on my chest, and sobbed.

It was all too much to handle. My husband hated the new foods I was making us eat (and he was still upset about the money I had wasted), my two children balked at every meal, and I had no idea what to cook. All of my go-to meals were gone. The anxiety and overwhelm felt like a heavy weight on my chest that I couldn't lift off.

At the end of the last chapter, in the Action Steps, I challenged you to go through your pantry and pull out food that contained gluten, dairy, soy, artificial flavors or colors, or excessive amounts of sugar. (If you haven't done this yet, grab a bookmark and go do it now!) What I DON'T want you to do is throw all that food away. You spent hard-earned money on that. There's no need to waste it.

Instead, make a list of all the foods you pulled from the pantry. Hang this list on your refrigerator. As you eat through each item on the list, mark it with a star. Then, each time you go shopping, look at the starred items on the list and instead of replacing them with the same item, replace them with a healthier alternative. To get you started, we've created a blank template for you to use. If you'd like to grab a copy, scan this QR code.

Are Gluten-Free Products Actually Healthier Alternatives?

"I'm just so disappointed." Katelynn's voice sounded angry, but her eyes told me what I already suspected. She wasn't so much angry as she was defeated, discouraged, and sad. She wanted the dietary changes she had already made to make the difference for her son, but she wasn't seeing the results she wanted to see.

"Everyone else has all these great stories of transformation. I just want to see some change in our family too."

Katelynn had been a part of my online program, the ADHD Thrive Method 4 Kids, for about two months. As a part of this program, caregivers can jump onto a Zoom call with me or one of my ADHD health coaches multiple times each week to talk through any obstacles they might be facing. This was Katelynn's first time joining us, and I saw the disappointment written all over her face.

"Tell me a little bit about what you're eating," I asked her.

"We've been gluten-, dairy-, soy-free for six weeks," she said. "One hundred percent. Our whole family has changed the way we eat, and I homeschool, so there's no way my son is sneaking food. We don't have anything for him to sneak in the house. And I'm always with him."

Sneaking food had been on my radar. It's unfortunately relatively common with children when we remove the foods they love and replace them with healthier alternatives. (Don't worry. We'll talk about how to deal with sneaking foods in a later chapter!) But for Katelynn, that wasn't the issue.

"What does a typical week look like?" I asked her. "Walk me through what you might normally eat for breakfast, lunch, dinner, and snacks."

THAT was the key. Katelynn had removed gluten, dairy, and soy from her family's diet, but she hadn't removed processed foods. She had replaced *gluten-filled* packaged foods with *gluten-free* packaged foods. For breakfast, they were eating gluten-free pancakes, waffles, or cereal. For lunch, gluten-free chicken nuggets most days, along with occasional hot dogs or frozen gluten-free and dairy-free pizza. Dinner was much of the same: packaged, quick convenience foods.

Unfortunately, packaged foods are still packaged foods, and they are not what our children's bodies need to reduce inflammation in the gut. It's not only about removing the inflammatory foods (though that is, of course, very important). It's also about replacing those foods with HEALTHY alternatives. So, what are those healthy alternatives? Let's dive in and see.

What to Eat

Because so many of the typical kid-friendly foods contain gluten, dairy, and soy, it can be challenging for caregivers to figure out what to feed their families. Many end up doing what Katelynn did: using a packaged item similar to the one they threw out. Unfortunately, as Katelynn learned, this doesn't typically create the kind of results people want to see.

What caregivers need to do instead is replace those packaged items with micronutrient-rich whole foods like the following:

- Vegetables (such as carrots, broccoli, cauliflower, spinach, kale, peppers, brussels sprouts, asparagus, green beans, etc.)

- Fruit (blueberries, raspberries, bananas, apples, grapes, blackberries, cherries, oranges, mangos, pears, etc.)
- Beans
- Eggs
- Grass-fed organic animal protein (such as beef, chicken, turkey, and collagen—we will take a look at this more in a later chapter)
- Wild-caught fish
- Nuts and seeds
- Gluten-free grains (such as quinoa, rice, and gluten-free oats)
- Healthy fats (such as avocado, olive, and coconut oil)

When I first changed our diet, I made it way too complicated. I tried to create these lavish meals with a ton of different ingredients, when really I needed to get back to nature. There's nothing wrong with a chicken breast, a side of sauteed broccoli and carrots, and sliced fruit. This simple meal is packed full of nutrients that our children need and, as a bonus, it's quick and easy. No culinary degree needed.

When planning meals, try to keep the packaged foods down to a minimum. What we can create in our own kitchens from real ingredients is always so much more nutritious than what we can buy at a store. Like Katelynn learned the hard way, it's not only about what you REMOVE from the diet but also about what you ADD. The more whole foods you provide for your family, the quicker you will likely see results.

But let's be honest. We're busy. I own a business, work from home, have two children, and participate in plenty of extracurricular activities. It's not always possible to cook everything from scratch. I don't want to spend all my extra time in the kitchen, and I'm guessing that unless you absolutely LOVE cooking, you don't either. Some packaged goods are necessary to maintain this healthy lifestyle.

I can hear the questions already: "You just said NOT to eat packaged foods and that if you just replace one packaged food for another, you'll never get to where you want to go. But now you're saying we can have packaged foods. What am I missing?"

The reality is, we are all busy families. If we could eat 100 percent whole foods and NO processed foods, that would be best, of course. But how realistic is that? For my family—and for most of the families I work with—that's not plausible.

The goal of the ADHD diet is a lifestyle change, and the only way this change is going to stick is if it's doable for you. For that reason, I tell my clients that it's all about balance. Try to make most of your meals from whole fruits, vegetables, and protein sources. But have some healthy, packaged items on hand for those days when you're too busy or too tired to cook.

When buying packaged items, the fewer ingredients, the better. If you can't pronounce or aren't familiar with an item on the ingredient list, then don't buy it. Only eat foods that you know all the ingredients for.

> **IF YOU CAN'T PRONOUNCE AN INGREDIENT ON A FOOD'S LABEL, DON'T PUT THAT FOOD IN YOUR CART. LEAVE IT ON THE SHELF.**

Going to the grocery store after cleaning out my kitchen was a daunting task. I felt incredibly unprepared. I knew a little bit—no gluten, dairy, or soy—but not enough to actually feel confident. To make this process easier for you, I put together a Kitchen Clean-Out Printable. It has 20 common products that can be found at most grocery stores, as well as 20 healthier alternatives. If you'd like to grab your printable, you can do that by scanning this QR code.

In the meantime, here are a few of my absolute favorite better-for-you alternatives.

DAIRY-FREE MILKS

Rice milk has a thin watery consistency and is light and naturally sweet. It is great on cereal and in cooking but might be a little watery for hot drinks.

Hemp milk is creamy, with a stronger robust flavor than any other dairy-free milk. It is great for cooking, especially savory dishes.

Oat milk is creamy and naturally sweet. It is great for cooking but too heavy for baking. Make sure that the oat milk you purchase is gluten-free, as not all of it is!

Almond milk has a slightly nutty flavor and is creamy. It is perfect for coffee or tea and in cooking and baking.

Hazelnut milk is light with a strong nutty flavor. It is great in drinks and light desserts but not great in cooking or baking.

Coconut milk is smooth, fresh and does not have a very strong flavor. It is similar to 2% dairy milk. It is ideal for all uses, especially in smoothies!

Cashew milk is smooth, creamy, slightly nutty, and sweet and is great for cooking, desserts and making cream.

Macadamia milk is high in healthy fats. Be sure to look for unsweetened macadamia milk as the other options tend to have high added sugars.

Gluten-Free Flours

Flour is a common ingredient in many foods such as bread, cookies, cakes, and pasta. There are three basic types of flour: light, medium, and heavy. Here are some of my favorites of each type:

- **Light flours (also known as starches)**—Light flours don't offer as much nutrition as other, heavier flours, but they are helpful for binding and creating the texture and structure that you would get with gluten. Some light flours to consider purchasing include arrowroot flour, corn starch, potato starch, and tapioca starch.

- **Medium flours**—Medium flours are more nourishing than light flours but are also denser. They become lighter and more stable when combined with a starch. Medium gluten-free flours include the following: fava bean flour, garbanzo bean/chickpea flour, millet flour, oat flour, quinoa flour, sorghum flour, and white rice flour.

- **Heavy flours**—The most nutrient dense flours, these are rarely used alone. When using heavy flours, it is best to mix them with a medium flour as well as a starch. Heavy flours include the following: almond flour, amaranth flour, brown rice flour, buckwheat flour, coconut flour, corn flour, and teff flour.[21]

When families first begin switching over to healthier alternatives, though, I often recommend they pick up a pre-made one-to-one all-purpose flour. These flours are typically made using a combination of light, medium, and heavy flours, making them ideal for baking. When using one-to-one gluten-free flour blends, many families can't even tell the difference between "regular" foods and gluten-free ones! When using one-to-one flours, you can typically substitute it one-to-one in any recipes that call for all-purpose flour.

Another option is to make your own flour blend, using a variety of the light, medium, and heavy flours. If you'd like three of my favorite DIY gluten-free flour blends, scan this QR code.

Label Reading 101

The most successful families I work with are those who are diligent about reading labels. The other day, one of the moms in my program vented in our private Facebook group: "I've been buying organic chia seeds for months, assuming they were free of all the ingredients we are supposed to avoid. I thought, *They're organic and they're seeds, so there's no way wheat could be in them!* Today, I pulled out the package and glanced at the ingredients: *May contain wheat!* WHAT?! Why would chia seeds contain wheat?"

She was flabbergasted. Sadly, I have learned the hard way that many foods that shouldn't contain wheat do (or include the warning "may contain," which is almost as bad). I cannot say enough about how important it is to read labels on every single item you buy. Most people are shocked when they realize how many of their pantry items contain gluten, dairy, or soy.

When looking at a food label, there is a significant amount of information included. Much of that information is helpful, but for our purposes in helping our children with ADHD, there are only three areas of the label that we need to focus on: the ingredient list, the amount of added sugar, and the allergen list.

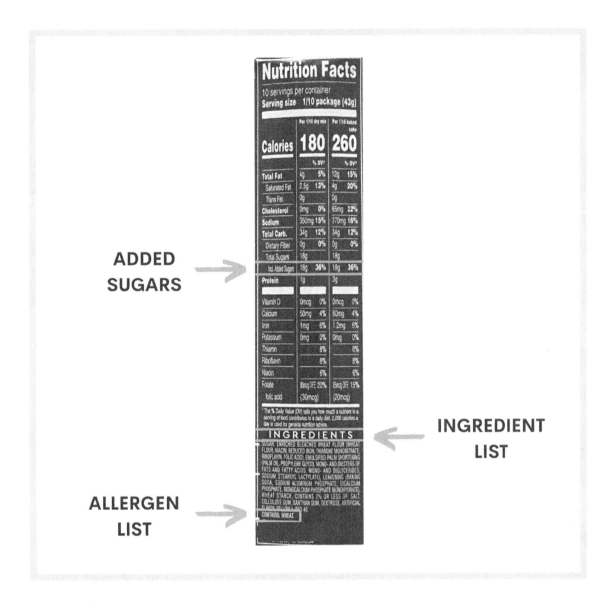

The allergen list will include any of the top eight allergens that are in the product. These top eight allergens include

- Milk
- Eggs
- Fish
- Crustacean shellfish

- Tree nuts
- Peanuts
- Wheat
- Soybeans

On first reading, then, it seems like this list should suffice for our purposes. If wheat, soy, and milk aren't listed in the allergen list, the product should be okay, right? Unfortunately, no. There are some gluten-containing grains that do not have to be listed on the allergen label—in particular, barley and rye. You might also remember that along with gluten, dairy, and soy, artificial flavors and colors are also very detrimental to our children with ADHD. That's why a simple reading of the allergen list is not enough. We need to dig a little bit deeper.

The next place to check is the ingredient list. As I said before, if there are ingredients you can't pronounce or don't know what they are, it's best to avoid that product. It's also best to avoid products that contain the items listed in Chapter 2. Remember, we can provide you with a list of products to avoid. Just scan this QR code.

The final thing to check before purchasing a product is the amount of added sugar. Children in this country eat WAY too much sugar. In order to help our children with ADHD become their best selves, we need to limit their sugar intake. As I mentioned earlier, the American Heart Association recommends that children eat less than 25 grams (6 teaspoons) of ADDED sugar daily. However, in my experience working with children with ADHD, this amount should be cut in half. Caregivers should aim to provide their children with less than 12 grams (3 teaspoons) of ADDED sugar daily.

Many find this surprisingly difficult to achieve, and it's really no wonder when you look at some of the foods we eat. For instance, I checked out the sugar content in a yogurt at the grocery store the other day (and it was even a "healthier" dairy-free option), and this tiny, 5-ounce container had 13 grams of added sugar in it. Thirteen grams! That's already MORE than the daily allotment for our children!

Ketchup also has a surprising amount of sugar in it. I looked up one popular brand, and it had 4 grams of added sugar in 1 tablespoon of ketchup. Barbecue sauce is even worse than ketchup, with a whopping 16 grams of added sugar per 2 tablespoons. Fruit juice, something many caregivers believe to be healthy for their children (side note: it's NOT!) has 26 grams of sugar in one 8-ounce cup. Even though this isn't added sugar (it's the sugar that comes naturally from fruit), this is still WAY too much for our children.

I haven't even touched on soda, which, depending on the brand you choose, can have 39, 46, or even 61 grams of added sugar per can! Is this shocking to anyone else? When I first realized just how much sugar American companies are adding to our food and drink supply, I was appalled. This needs to change! We are creating sugar addicts, and many of us don't even realize it.

Now that you know the truth and understand how to read labels, you have the opportunity to be part of the change. As I said before, the food and drink industry might not listen to our voices, but they will listen to our money. If enough of us refuse to buy products with excessive amounts of sugar added, we will change the landscape. Companies won't keep making products that aren't being sold.

What About "May Contain . . ." or "Made in a Facility That . . ."?

As you begin reading labels, you'll likely run across a warning label that reads, "May contain …" or "Made in a facility that processes …" or "Made on shared equipment that processes …" Caregivers in my program are often unsure about these products. If the allergen label, ingredient list, and amounts of added sugars are okay, are products with one of these warnings okay to eat, or do they need to be avoided?

This is a great question. Unfortunately, the answer isn't clear-cut. If a product says "May contain …," it's best to avoid that product. Studies[22] have shown that when products say "May contain …," they often DO contain, so steer clear of any products with this particular warning label.

The other two warnings ("Made in a facility …" and "Made on shared equipment …"), though, are not as black and white as the "May contain …" warning. If a child doesn't have a significant allergy to a product listed on these warnings, I typically advise that it's okay to eat this product if the other parts of the label (the ingredient list and sugar content) look okay.

> PLEASE NOTE, WE'RE NOT TALKING ABOUT TRUE ALLERGIES HERE. IF YOU OR YOUR CHILD HAS A TRUE ALLERGY TO A CERTAIN FOOD, YOU'LL NEED TO CONSULT WITH YOUR DOCTOR ABOUT WHICH FOODS YOU CAN AND CAN NOT HAVE.

When it comes to the "Made in a facility ..." and "Made on shared equipment ..." labels, it's all about balance. You have to balance convenience and budget with health and do what's best for your family. Of course, if you're able to avoid products with any of these warnings, that's the best-case scenario. Not all families are able to do this. Do what's doable for you!

That doesn't mean, however, that you can eat a little bit of gluten here or there! Families who continue to have gluten in their diets don't make the progress they want to make. This just means that if you have to eat a product whose label says it was made in a facility that also processes wheat, you don't need to stress over this.

In summary, pay attention to the three critical aspects of the label: the ingredient list, the sugar content, and the allergen list. Avoid products that contain gluten, dairy, soy, or artificial flavors or colors. Also avoid products that state they "May contain ..." these offenders. But don't stress over the "Made in a facility ..." and "Made on shared equipment ..." labels.

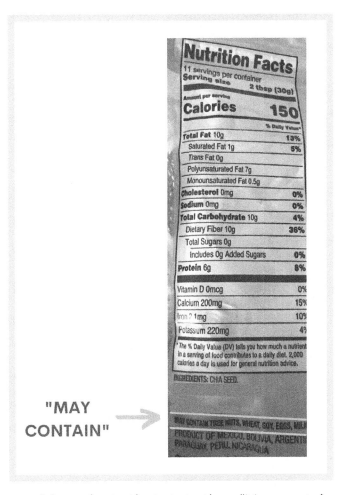

Water, Water Everywhere!

One final note before we close out this chapter on what TO eat: water is vital in the healing journey. Water carries nutrients to cells, helps the body flush out waste, enables the body to dissolve minerals so they are accessible throughout, and carries out a variety of other important functions.[23] It also aids in detoxification, which is critical for our children with compromised systems.

According to the American Academy of Pediatrics, "Children ages 1–3 years need approximately 4 cups of beverages per day ... This increases for older kids to around 5 cups for 4–8 year-olds, and 7–8 cups for older children."[24]

So, how can you get your children to drink water, without it becoming *another* thing they fight with you over? Here are some tips that work well for my family and the families with whom I work:

- **Take water with you everywhere you go.**

    Not only will this save you money (and keep you healthier) since you won't be grabbing a soda at a local gas station or convenience store, but it will also keep hydration at top of mind. Some families do this by keeping a fridge right next to their garage door. As they walk to their car, they grab a bottle of water each time. Other families would rather not use bottled water, so they have designated cups for each family member that they keep within reach at all times.

- **Use a fun cup.**

    There's just something about a fun cup that makes drinking water so much easier. Consider a small cup for your children, as it will fit better in their hands. I would also recommend allowing your children to pick out their own cups. This will help get buy-in from them and make them more likely to use the cups on a regular basis.

- **Use a straw.**

    Drinking through a straw enables you to drink large amounts of water faster. Don't believe it? Give it a try and see for yourself. In both my own experience and in the experience of the families I work with, drinking water from a straw equates to more water consumed.

- **Add fresh fruit or veggies, such as strawberries, lemons, or cucumbers.**

    One of the reasons many of our kids don't drink water is because of its bland taste. Add fresh fruit to give it a splash of flavor. You could even freeze these fruits in ice cube trays to add to your glasses. My favorites to enhance taste are strawberries, pineapple chunks, lemons, and cucumbers.

- **Buy tiny cups or bottles.**

    Not only do these smaller cups fit in a child's hands better, but they're also fun! Consider having a challenge to see who can drink the most tiny cups of water each day.

- **Consider a reward system.**

    When your children reach a certain goal, they get stickers. Once they receive a certain number of stickers, they get a reward. Though there are pros and cons to using a reward system, it can be a good way to build a habit. Many caregivers find that once they create that habit of drinking more water, they don't have to continue using the reward system long-term.

- **Set a good example.**

    Our kids aren't going to want water if we are constantly downing soda, tea, or coffee. Think about your own experiences. If you are with someone who is drinking your favorite drink, would you continue to drink water as you sat with them over breakfast, or would you want to follow their example and order yourself a delicious (albeit bad for you) drink? Many of us—myself included—would ditch the water. It's hard to drink something healthy when those around you splurge on a treat. Our children are the same. They will follow our example, not our advice.

- **Don't offer other things to drink.
    If you don't buy it, they won't drink it.**

    Many caregivers, when they first begin working with me, are worried about their children not drinking milk anymore. They are especially concerned about calcium. But the truth is, children don't really need milk. There are other ways to get the calcium they need. Here are a few of my favorites:

> ## Calcium-Rich Foods
>
> - Fortified almond milk and rice milk
> - Canned pink salmon with edible bones
> - Sweet potatoes
> - Gluten-free oatmeal
> - Veggies such as cooked broccoli, Chinese cabbage, and acorn squash
> - Papaya, dried figs, and oranges
> - Greens such as turnip, collard greens, or kale
> - Beans such as garbanzo, kidney, navy, and even canned baked beans
> - Seeds such as chia seeds, sunflower seeds, and sesame seeds
> - Canned shrimp
> - Canned sardines

- **Our children also don't need fruit juice.**

    Fruit juice is often chock-full of sugar. It's much better to get nutrients from fresh fruit instead of fruit juice. Stick with water or smoothies for your children's beverages, and they are sure to drink more water because they won't be full on other drinks.

Remember: if you don't have it in the house, they won't eat or drink it!

The Way Out

Two weeks after my kitchen raid, I landed on my bedroom floor, on the verge of a panic attack because of the changes I had made. Too fast. With too little support. And all alone. I don't suggest you do what I did. Take it slow. Make one small change a day, or even one small change a week.

I tell all the families I work with that Rome wasn't built in a day. It's not necessary to make all of these changes at once. Look over the action steps at the end of this chapter to remind yourself of what you will be working toward, but DON'T STRESS!

Remember: one step forward is still a step in the right direction. You've got this!

Note: If, after reading this chapter, you feel that you could benefit from additional support, I would be happy to chat with you about how to implement these changes. My team and I offer a free ADHD Thrive Breakthrough Call. You can set up that free call by scanning the QR code at the end of this chapter.

Chapter Highlights

- What we create in our own kitchens from real ingredients is always so much more nutritious than what we can buy at a store. Packaged foods are not what our children's bodies need to reduce inflammation.

- It's not only about what you REMOVE from the diet but also about what you ADD. Try to eat MOSTLY whole, micronutrient-dense fruits, veggies, protein sources, and healthy fats, and save those packaged foods for those instances when you really need them.

- When buying packaged foods, choose healthier alternatives. The fewer ingredients, the better. Don't buy anything if it contains an ingredient you can't pronounce or aren't familiar with.

- Make sure to read every single label! Pay special attention to the following sections on the label: the allergen warning, the ingredient list, and the sugar content.

- Avoid products that state they "May contain ..." gluten, dairy, or soy.

- Encourage your child to drink as much water as possible. Aim for 4 cups per day for children aged one to three, 5 cups for children aged four to eight, and 7–8 cups for older children.

Action Steps

1. Make a list of all the foods you pulled from the pantry that contain gluten, dairy, soy, excessive sugar, or artificial flavors or colors. Hang this list on your refrigerator. As you eat through each item on the list, mark it with a star. Then, each time you go shopping, look at the starred items on the list and instead of replacing them with the same item, replace them with a healthier alternative. To get you started, we've created a blank template for you to use. You can grab that template, as well as our favorite gluten-free flour recipes and our Kitchen Clean-Out Printable by scanning this QR code.

2. Choose ten foods in your pantry. Look at the labels and see if there are any ingredients you can't pronounce or you don't know what they are. Use this action step to practice your label-reading skills.

3. Start looking at labels every time you shop. Only buy products that are gluten-, dairy-, or soy-free. Also avoid artificial flavors and colors. Keep an eye on those added sugars and the "May contain …" warnings!

4. Choose one of the tips (or several) to help your child drink more water.

5. If, after reading this chapter, you feel like you could benefit from additional support, I would be happy to chat with you about how to implement these changes. My team and I offer a free ADHD Thrive Breakthrough Call. Sign up for that free call by scanning this QR code.

CHAPTER 4:

Superfoods

Sometimes, superfoods aren't so super.

Did I get your attention? Maybe you had to read that first sentence a couple of times. After all, why would I devote an entire chapter to superfoods if they aren't that great?

What I mean is, no one food can serve as the be-all and end-all for a nutritious lifestyle. Our bodies are meant to have variety. One of the moms I worked with recently, Angie, learned this the hard way.

We were on a weekly Zoom call, and Angie was thrilled because her daughter was finally eating something other than cereal for breakfast.

"My daughter really likes her routines," Angie said. "But I think I've found a way to use them to my advantage! She used to eat cereal every day, but I've finally got her switched over to cinnamon blueberry oatmeal!"

Angie's eyes sparkled with excitement. I really didn't want to burst her bubble. She seemed so happy. *How can I let her down gently?* I thought to myself.

I waited a few moments and then asked, "Does she eat that every day?"

Angie affirmed my suspicions by saying proudly, "Yep, every day."

I explained to Angie that unfortunately, even eating the healthiest foods (if we eat the same food each day) can do damage to our children's compromised bodies.

Do you remember reading about leaky gut in Chapter 1? When someone has a leaky gut, the foods they eat most often are the ones that are most likely to leak out of the gut lining, leading to an inflammatory response in the body.

What that means is, if we give our children the same foods each day—even healthy foods—those foods are the ones their bodies will likely develop a sensitivity to. Angie was inadvertently creating an opportunity for a new food sensitivity to develop.

What I challenged her to do is to get her daughter to eat food on a rotational basis. Don't let her eat the same foods every day, but rather eat them every three or four days. By rotating foods, we are doing two things: 1) we are guaranteeing that our bodies get a variety of foods and, thus, a variety of nutrients, and 2) if leaky gut is a concern, we are making it less likely for the same foods to leak through the gut and create inflammatory responses.

Angie got one thing right: she was providing a nutritious breakfast for her daughter. Blueberries make the top of the list as far as antioxidant content goes. They also lower blood pressure, lower cholesterol, and combat inflammation and are rich in nutrients such as potassium, vitamin C, and fiber.

Angie chose a great fruit for her daughter to eat. Oats are also a great choice, as they are packed with nutrients our bodies need, and Angie did well to get certified gluten-free oats too! She did several things correctly. What she failed to do, though, was offer other amazing foods to her daughter.

In the pages ahead, we're going to look at some of the foods I suggested Angie introduce into her daughter's diet. Let's jump in.

What Are Superfoods?

The term "superfood" has become a well-known word, but most people don't really know how to define it. Hopefully, by the end of this chapter, you will be fully versed on what superfoods are, as well as have a running list of foods to try moving forward!

All superfoods have the following in common: they contain a high concentration of vitamins and minerals without packing on too many calories. To be classified as a superfood, a food must have three things: 1) high nutrient density per serving, 2) high nutrient diversity (meaning that there are lots of different nutrients in the food, rather than just a surplus of one nutrient), and 3) the absence of toxins. All superfoods have a high concentration and variety of:

- Vitamins
- Minerals
- Antioxidants
- Phytonutrients
- Fiber
- Healthy fats
- Quality protein

Superfoods do NOT have the following:

- Added sugars
- Artificial ingredients
- Harmful toxins

If you search online for the "top superfoods," you will likely find many different foods listed on each website you visit, and these lists will probably vary from site to site. Therefore, the list that follows isn't meant to be exhaustive. Rather, it includes some of my favorites that I suggested Angie begin incorporating into her family's meals on a rotational basis.

The BEST Superfoods

- **Kale**—Kale is one of the most nutritious greens available. It is rich in antioxidants and high in fiber, calcium, iron, vitamin K, vitamin A, and vitamin C. Kale is also low in calories and very versatile. I love to hide kale in the smoothies I make for my children. I also mix it into salads and add it to stir-fry dishes.

- **Nuts**—Nuts are also very versatile. They can be added to trail mixes, eaten alone, thrown on top of yogurt for an added crunch, mixed into smoothies or salads, or crafted into nut butter. One of my favorite nuts is the almond. Almonds are chock-full of unsaturated fats (good fats), antioxidants, dietary fiber, phosphorus, potassium, magnesium, calcium, iron, and vitamin E.

- **Quinoa**—Quinoa contains all nine essential amino acids. These essential amino acids cannot be produced in the body by itself, so quinoa is a great way to obtain them all! It is also a great source of fiber with 6 grams per cup, and it's naturally gluten-free and simple to prepare.

- **Beans**—Beans pack the protein punch. In fact, just a half cup of beans has 7 grams of protein, which is the same as in 1 ounce of meat! Beans aid in digestion and help with balancing blood sugar. They are a heart-healthy snack and nutrient powerhouses, providing our bodies with zinc, iron, magnesium, and phosphorus. They, like some of the other superfoods previously listed, are also very versatile. Serve them as a main dish, a side dish, an appetizer, a snack, or even a dessert. My children LOVE the black bean chocolate muffins that I bake for them!

- **Blueberries**—As noted, blueberries are an amazing superfood. They are packed full of nutrients and can be served alone, in baked goods, in smoothies or salads, or even in salsa.

- **Eggs**—Eggs have gotten a bad reputation in recent years because of their cholesterol content, but the truth is that many studies confirm that eggs are, in fact, a superfood packed full of fiber and other nutrients our bodies need. One egg contains more than 20 percent of our daily need for vitamin D. Eggs also contain antioxidants and choline. Choline is crucial for brain cell structure and how the brain communicates with the rest of the body. Thinking back to Chapter 1 and the connection between the gut and brain, you can understand why eggs can be very beneficial for children with ADHD. Eggs also contain fiber, amino acids, vitamins A, B12, B2, and B5, iron, and phosphorus.

- **Salmon**—Salmon is rich in omega-3 fatty acids. These fatty acids strengthen cardiovascular health, immunity, eyesight, skin health, and longevity. For our children with ADHD, salmon is especially beneficial because of the way it improves brain function.

- **Gluten-free oats**—Oats are a naturally gluten-free super grain. They are affordable, easy to prepare, and a rockstar breakfast. They are high in fiber, boost energy levels, can be eaten hot or cold, and are versatile. Many of the families I work with add nuts or fruit or honey to their oatmeal. Many of them eat overnight oats on a rotational basis. They use oats for cookies, cakes, pancakes, gluten-free bread, and a variety of other dishes.

  Keep in mind: It's very important to buy certified gluten-free oats. That's because oats, though naturally free of gluten, are one of the foods most commonly contaminated with gluten. I have worked with many families who weren't making the progress they were hoping to make until they swapped out their regular oats for certified gluten-free ones.

- **Green tea**—Move over, milk, and make room for green tea! Green tea is loaded with antioxidants and is one of the healthiest beverages out there. Green tea also contains L-theanine, which is an amino acid that can help people feel calmer, improve attention span and focus, and support restful sleep. Because these are often areas of concern for our children with ADHD, green tea can be a great superfood (or in this case, superdrink) to add to your rotation.

- **Avocados**—Did you know that avocados are actually considered berries? It's true, and, as a berry, they are chock-full of many nutrients your body needs, such as vitamins C, K, E, and B6. Avocados also contain a large amount of healthy fats that keep us fuller longer and help to regulate blood-sugar levels. They are high in fiber too, resulting in better digestion and detoxification. Avocados are great in smoothies because they give them a nice, creamy texture without affecting the taste.

- **Pumpkin**—Pumpkin is especially rich in vitamin A, coming in at over 200 percent of our daily nutritional need in only one cup. Its high content of vitamin A, paired with other vitamins it provides, such as vitamin C, vitamin E, iron, and folate, help provide a huge immunity boost for those who eat it.

- **Flax seeds**—I love flax seeds, primarily because of the amount of omega-3 fatty acids they contain. Flax seeds are also a great source of plant-based protein. When children with ADHD consume them, they feel fuller longer.

- **Broccoli**—Broccoli is rich in vitamins C and K but also has anti-inflammatory properties, which is why I love encouraging families of children with ADHD to include this vegetable in their family's diet. The more the inflammation is reduced, the quicker they begin to see symptoms disappear.

- **Garlic**—Garlic, like many of these other superfoods, is a known immunity booster. Garlic has been used for quite some time to help with various medical conditions. Eating garlic might also help detoxify heavy metals (lead, for example) from the body.[25]

- **Lentils**—Lentils are edible seeds. They are rich in B vitamins, as well as iron, magnesium, potassium, and folate. Lentils are also an amazing source of plant-based protein and, because of their high fiber content, also support healthy gut bacteria.

- **Ginger**—People have been using ginger since ancient times for medicinal purposes. It is still a common home remedy for upset stomachs or nausea. Ginger aids in digestion and reduces inflammation, which is one of the primary reasons I love it for children with ADHD, who typically have significant inflammation in their bodies that can contribute to their symptoms.

- **Wheatgrass**—Many people on gluten-free diets avoid wheatgrass because they assume it contains gluten. Though wheatgrass does come from wheat, it is, in fact, gluten-free if harvested before it goes to seed. The grass of wheat does not contain gluten, just the seeds. Wheatgrass typically comes in juice form, though it can also be powdered. It is rich in antioxidants and is known for its anti-inflammatory and antibacterial properties. It also aids in detoxification and can improve brain function.

- **Acai berries**—Acai berries are rich in antioxidants (specifically anthocyanin), leading many researchers to believe that acai berries boost cognitive function by lowering oxidative stress and inflammation in the brain.

- **Goji berries**—Goji berries help stabilize blood sugar by balancing glucose and insulin levels in the blood.[26] They can also help with sleep and reduce feelings of depression and anxiety.[27] As many children with ADHD struggle with these things, goji berries are especially beneficial for them.

- **Honey**—Honey, like both ginger and garlic, has been used for thousands of years for medicinal purposes. You've probably heard of honey being used as a cough remedy, but it has several other health benefits too. It is rich in antioxidants, which help reduce oxidative stress inside the body.

  Keep in mind: though honey does have many amazing benefits, it is also high in natural sugar. Though a much better option than store-bought, processed table sugar, honey in excess is still not a good idea.

- **Cacao**—Cacao is rich in theobromine, and, as such, helps reduce inflammation in the body. Cacao is also a mood-boosting food, known to reduce depression and improve mood.

- **Maca**—Maca, or maca root, is a cruciferous vegetable related to kale, broccoli, and cauliflower. Maca root grows underground and looks like a turnip. Maca is loaded with vitamins and minerals and contains 20 amino acids. It provides vitamins B1, B6, B2, C, and E. Maca, like cacao, is also a mood booster. Many children with ADHD struggle with mood regulation, so adding foods like cacao and maca to their diets can be very beneficial.

- **Cinnamon**—Cinnamon can help regulate blood sugar, reduce inflammation, and improve brain function. Many people don't realize there are actually two types of cinnamon: Ceylon and cassia cinnamon. Most cinnamon that is in our supermarkets is cassia cinnamon. It is relatively easy to find and inexpensive. Ceylon cinnamon, in contrast, is more expensive but also much healthier. Cassia cinnamon contains coumarin, which can be toxic in large quantities. Ceylon cinnamon only contains a negligible amount and is therefore safer to consume regularly.

- **Almonds**—I mentioned almonds earlier in this chapter, but they deserve a section all to themselves. Almonds are a great source of healthy fat. They also contain fiber, protein, magnesium, and vitamin E. They are a great source of antioxidants and can help the body feel fuller longer, making them an excellent snack for children and adults alike.

- **Coconut**—Coconut is rich in copper, iron, and manganese. It is also a good protein source. One of the primary benefits of coconut is that it provides the body with fat. Contrary to popular belief, fat—in and of itself—is not a bad thing, especially for developing children. Our brains need fat to function at their best. Coconut can be an excellent source of fat for children.

SUPERFOODS

 KALE   BROCCOLI

 NUTS   GARLIC

 QUINOA   LENTILS

 BEANS   GINGER

 BLUEBERRIES   WHEATGRASS

 EGGS   ACAI BERRIES

 SALMON   GOJI BERRIES

 GF OATS   HONEY

 GREEN TEA   CACAO

 AVOCADOS   MACA

 PUMPKIN   CINNAMON

 FLAX SEEDS   ALMONDS

 COCONUT

What About Collagen and Protein Powders?

Other favorite staples of mine are collagen powder and protein powder. Proteins contain long chains of amino acids and are the building blocks of every cell. A complete protein is made of at least nine essential amino acids that can only be obtained from diet. Our bodies cannot synthesize them on their own. These complete proteins are found in foods derived from animals, such as meat, fish, and eggs.

Collagen, though similar in appearance to complete protein, is actually a different type of protein. It is not complete, meaning it does not have all nine essential amino acids. Instead, it is composed of nonessential amino acids that many of us are lacking.

Most children, and adults for that matter, are not getting enough protein or collagen from their diets, so adding in protein and collagen powders is often beneficial for the entire family. Between collagen powder and protein powder, which is better? Actually, both. Our bodies need both types of protein, so I typically suggest that families rotate: one day using collagen, the next using a complete protein powder, and so on. Variety is key to a healthy body!

Protein from an animal source helps to build and repair every structure in the body, whereas collagen protein is important because it is like a "glue" that holds the body together. Many people are aware of the amazing benefits of collagen powder for the skin, hair, and nails, but did you know that collagen is also beneficial for the gut barrier? The gut barrier, as we have already discussed, is often broken down in children with ADHD, so collagen can play an important piece in rebuilding that gut barrier. It's also beneficial for bones and connective tissues and helps them stay strong, healthy, and flexible.

Collagen production rapidly declines after the age of 40. This results in wrinkles, thinning bones, weaker joints, and thinning hair. It negatively impacts many aspects of our health and vitality.

An additional benefit of collagen powder is that it keeps the body feeling full longer. Many parents have told me that when they introduced collagen powder into their children's diets, their children complained less often of being hungry. Remember to buy collagen powder from a reputable source and ensure it is gluten-, dairy-, and soy-free. My absolute favorite collagen powders come from grass-fed animals and are free of GMOs, antibiotics, hormones, and fillers. Steer clear of those with additives or additional ingredients. Collagen is great to add to coffee, tea, broths, soups, or smoothies.

Getting Superfoods into Our SuperKids

I can hear the objections already: "That's great, Dana, but my child would NEVER eat kale or salmon or wheatgrass!" It can certainly be difficult to get a picky eater to try some of these superfoods. It's one thing to get them to eat blueberries, but kale or wheatgrass? That's a whole different ball game!

So how do you get your little one to eat these superfoods? In the next few pages, I'm going to share some of my best tips and tricks to incorporate superfoods into the diet of even the pickiest of eaters.

Tip #1: SNEAK Them In

One of the best ways to get superfoods into children's diets is by sneaking them in. Many of these superfoods (such as kale, nuts, avocados, pumpkin, and flax seeds) can easily be added to smoothies without changing the flavor at all. Honey can be added to smoothies to give them a little bit of extra sweetness. You can also drizzle honey on top of fresh fruit. To add veggies (broccoli, for instance) into the diet of a child who doesn't like them, I puree them and then add them to spaghetti sauce. I have pureed zucchini, squash, peppers, and a variety of other veggies and added them to sauces and soups without my children having any idea.

Many of these superfoods can easily be added to baked goods too. Flax seeds, for example, as well as powdered green tea and garbanzo bean flour, can all be added to baked goods with very little change in texture, taste, or appearance. The key is to add small amounts of the superfood to begin with, so that the taste isn't noticeable.

Tip #2: SWAP Them Out

Many families I work with already use several superfoods, but they don't buy the best varieties. For instance, most regularly use chocolate chips in their baking but might not use ones that are at least 70 percent cocoa. Swap out the unhealthy alternative for the superfood version of chocolate chips. When shopping for these, make sure the product you grab is a dairy-free version.

When buying honey, buy the raw variety instead of the more processed one. When buying cinnamon, opt for the Ceylon instead of the cassia variety that is found at most supermarkets. When buying oats, make sure they are gluten-free. Take a second look at each of the foods listed in this chapter and think about which ones you could easily sneak into foods you are currently eating and which ones you could easily swap out for better alternatives.

Tip #3: Be SILLY

"You're not getting up from this table until you take at least one bite."

The rest of the family was done eating, but not eight-year-old Sam. He remained where he was, arms crossed in front of his chest, lip slightly pouty, a look of determination in his eyes. He was nothing if not persistent. When he set his mind to something, there was little that would make him change it. This particular evening, his mind was set on not putting the blueberry into his mouth. No matter what his mom said.

And his mom said plenty. She threatened him. "No TV for the rest of the night if you don't finish your dinner." She encouraged him. "You can do it, Son. It's just one little berry." She begged him. "Come on, please." None of these strategies worked.

"The next two hours, he and I argued back and forth, but he still refused to eat it. Once bath time came around, I finally gave up." His mom, Rachel, recounted the story for me a few days after it had happened.

How often do your mealtimes go a similar way? So many families of children with ADHD struggle with meals at the table. Take a look at the list below and think about whether your family dinners have any of these elements:

- Children who can't stay seated or sit still
- Children who refuse to let other people talk and interrupt incessantly
- Arguments
- Complaints about the food on the table
- Irritability

One tip that our families find very helpful when attempting to introduce superfoods into the diet is to make mealtime fun. When children enjoy mealtimes, they are more likely to eat the foods put in front of them. So, how can you make them fun? Here are some ideas:

Game #1: Guess What's in My Smoothie

Play a game of Guess What's in My Smoothie. To do this, add all sorts of superfoods into your child's smoothie—without them watching—and then encourage them to guess each ingredient. Not only is this fun, but it's also a great way to encourage children to drink more of their smoothie and get more of those great nutrients into their bodies.

Game #2: Superfood Family Challenge

Another way to make eating superfoods fun is to do a family food challenge. To do this, introduce one superfood a week. Each night at dinner, everyone in the family takes at least one bite of the new food. Once the bites are taken, a checkmark is added to a chart. Once the family reaches the end of the week and has a certain number of checkmarks, the entire family gets a reward that everyone will enjoy.

One question I get asked often by families who are just beginning this journey is whether everyone in the family needs to adjust their diets. In my experience, when everyone is on board and making the changes together, it makes the entire journey much easier for the child. That way, the child does not feel singled out or like there is something wrong with him or her. Every family has to decide for themselves if this is the direction they want to go, but it's definitely my recommendation. Especially with challenges like this, getting the entire family involved makes the game more fun and the child more likely to cooperate.

Game #3: Eat the Rainbow

You've likely heard the saying "Eat the rainbow." It's excellent advice, but it can also be turned into a game. To play this game, draw a blank rainbow on a large piece of paper. Every member of the family gets a copy of this blank rainbow. As the game progresses, children get to color the rainbow as they eat foods in that color. For instance, if a child eats kale, they get to color the GREEN arch. If the child eats pumpkin, they get to color the ORANGE arch, and so on. The first person who fills up their rainbow for the day wins.

My team and I have created a Rainbow Template for you to play this game. You can grab it by scanning this QR code.

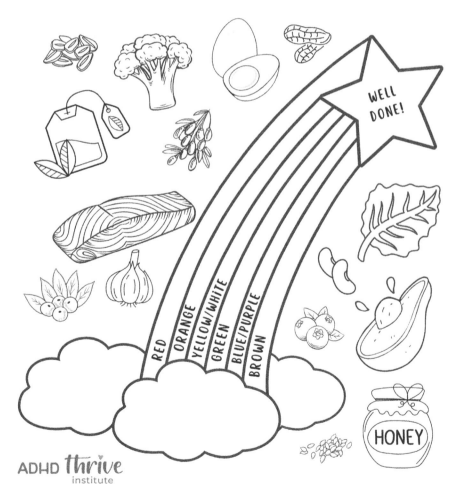

Tip #4: Try SUPERFOOD Blends

One final way that I love getting a surplus of superfoods into the diet is to invest in a superfood blend. These powders can be added to water, smoothies, or even baked goods or sauces. Make sure when you are choosing one, that you choose a clean brand with no additives or extra nasties.

Take a look at some of the ingredients in a superfood blend that I have at my home: kale, broccoli, spirulina, turmeric, ginger, wheatgrass, elderberry, cherry, and more. By adding clean superfood powders to your regular rotation of foods, you are able to pack the nutritional punch big-time.

The Rest of Angie's Story

Angie's face sank when she realized that even though blueberries and oatmeal were better than cereal, they still shouldn't be eaten every day. As hard as I tried to break that news gently, she was nonetheless discouraged.

"Back to square one, I guess." She shrugged her shoulders and looked away from the screen.

I told Angie all about the Eat the Rainbow game, the Guess What's in My Smoothie game, and the Superfood Family Challenge. As I spoke, I saw the hope begin to ignite in her eyes again. I asked her to pick one of the three games. She chose Guess What's in My Smoothie.

The next week, she joined our Group Coaching Call and filled me in on her progress.

"You'll never believe it! I put kale in her smoothie. Kale! And even when she guessed it, she wasn't disgusted. She was having so much fun with the game that we played it every day last week." Angie successfully added the following superfoods to her daughter's smoothies in just one week: pumpkin, oats, kale, flax seeds, green tea, cinnamon, honey, almonds, black beans, and broccoli.

There is no one superfood that can provide the body with all the nutrients it needs to function at its best. Still, there's a reason they're called SUPERfoods. When someone eats a variety of them, they really are super and can do amazing things in the body: from boosting the immune system to improving gut function to regulating mood, and more.

Chapter Highlights

- It's important to rotate foods, ensuring you don't eat the same foods every day. Variety is key.

- Superfoods are a vital part of naturally reducing ADHD symptoms. By incorporating these superfoods into our children's diets, we are providing them with exactly the nutrients their bodies need to rebuild.

- Sometimes, it takes a little bit of creativity to get children to eat superfoods, especially those that aren't as "kid-friendly," such as kale or wheatgrass.

- Try the following strategies to incorporate more superfoods into your family's diet: 1) SNEAK them in, 2) SWAP them out, 3) be SILLY, and 4) try SUPERFOOD blends.

Action Steps

1. Look over the list of superfoods in this chapter one more time
2. Choose one superfood you can SNEAK in
3. Choose one superfood you can SWAP out
4. Choose one way you will be SILLY with superfoods this week
5. Consider adding SUPERFOOD powders to your weekly rotation of meals
6. If you'd like a copy of the Rainbow Template, scan this QR code

CHAPTER 5:

GMOs and Organic Produce— What Caregivers Need to Know

If you're looking for controversy, you've come to the right place. Controversy consistently surrounds the topic of GMOs. Are they good or bad? Do they help the farmer or hurt the consumer? Are they dangerous to eat or completely safe? In the pages ahead, we're going to evaluate the research on GMOs, both the benefits and the dangers.

But first, let's seek to understand what GMOs are.

What Are GMOs?

GMO stands for genetically modified organism. GMOs are living organisms whose genetic material has been artificially manipulated in a lab setting. This is done through genetic engineering when plant, animal, bacteria, or virus genes are combined in a way that does not naturally occur otherwise.

Farmers have been modifying plants for thousands of years through selective breeding and cross-breeding. As you can imagine, this is a relatively slow way to modify plants and animals. Genetic modification, however, is much quicker and more targeted. It has only been around since the 1980s, when the first GMO product entered the market: insulin for diabetes.

In 1994, the FDA approved the first GMO tomato, claiming it was just as safe as those traditionally bred. Following the tomato came other GMO plants: summer squash, soybeans, cotton, corn, papayas, potatoes, and canola. In 2005, alfalfa and sugar beets were added to this list of GMO products. Then, ten years later, a genetically modified salmon was released into the market. Finally, in 2017, apples were added to the list of GMOs. You might have noticed in recent years the term "bioengineered" on some food labels. That's because in 2016, Congress passed a law requiring *some* foods to feature this particular label.[28]

GMOs are created using four steps: 1) identify the appealing gene in the original organism, 2) copy the information from that gene, 3) insert that genetic information into another organism, and 4) grow a new organism. It sounds simple when boiled down to these four steps, but it's quite the scientific process and definitely something that cannot occur naturally.

The Pros

Most GMOs fall into one of two categories: herbicide tolerant or pesticide producing. Herbicide-tolerant plants can withstand herbicide so the farmer can kill weeds without hurting the plant. Pesticide-producing plants produce their own pesticides, so the farmer doesn't have to spray them. This is definitely one benefit of GMOs, as farmers are able to significantly reduce their use of chemical insecticides.

One family in Bangladesh saw their yearly income double when they introduced the *Bacillus thuringiensis* (Bt) eggplant—which was the first genetically modified organism in South Asia—to their family farm.[29] The Bt eggplant was genetically modified in such a way that farmers were able to significantly reduce the use of pesticides, thus creating higher yield with fewer chemicals and less cost involved.

Many farmers, especially those in lower-income countries, work without protective shoes, glasses, or clothing. The constant onslaught of chemicals from pesticides often makes these farmers sick. By using GMO seeds, these farmers can reduce or completely eliminate the use of dangerous pesticides.

From a farmer's perspective, GMOs seem health-conscious, convenient, and efficient. After all, when utilizing GMOs, farmers are able to produce more plants with fewer resources, protecting themselves from harmful pesticides in the process, and saving them money and time. There are fewer crops destroyed by insects or weeds. They often have high crop yield, equating to more income. It seems like a win-win.

The Cons

But is it possible there's more to the story than this? Unfortunately, GMOs are a manipulation of nature, and the long-term consequences of their use are still unknown. As noted, GMOs only entered the scene in the 1980s and didn't become widespread in our food supply until the 1990s, so we really don't know how consuming them is going to affect our health long-term. We also don't know how they will affect our planet or our animals.

Remember, GMOs are, in essence, manufactured plants. They can't be found in nature ANYWHERE. They are created in labs and then pushed on consumers, many times without our knowledge.

GMOs are created for a number of reasons, including, as mentioned previously, the ability to withstand herbicide or insecticide application. And as mentioned, when GMOs are pesticide-producing, farmers are able to reduce or even eliminate their usage of pesticides. Most would agree this is a good thing. But what about herbicide-tolerant GMOs?

Because plants are herbicide tolerant, some farmers actually use MORE herbicides because the herbicides no longer hurt their crops. They kill the weeds alone. That means that though we might be reducing the amount of insecticides because of GMOs, we are actually increasing the amount of herbicides.[30]

Have you heard of glyphosate? Glyphosate is one of the most widely used herbicides in the world. Studies have suggested that glyphosate is a probable carcinogen.[31] With the introduction and widespread use of GMOs, our country is now flooded with carcinogenic weed killers. I think we can all agree this is a major concern with GMOs.

Along with herbicide-tolerant and pesticide-producing GMOs, other GMOs are created to ensure a longer shelf life. Though I can understand why the food industry would like to increase shelf life (more profit, of course), I have to wonder what benefit a longer shelf life is to the consumer. Sure, I guess that means we can buy produce and it won't get moldy for weeks, thus enabling us to shop less often and have food that lasts longer in our fridges.

But is that really what we want? A tomato that won't go bad for weeks? My rule of thumb is that if something doesn't spoil, it's probably WAY too processed! Though I can understand a consumer's desire to make their produce last longer, is it worth the cost to our health? To me, it's not. I would rather have to shop more often for my produce and KNOW it's not dangerous for my family, than to shop less often but remain unsure of the damage to our health.

At this time, there is a lot of consumer doubt, confusion, and issues within the GMO industry. In the United States, three federal agencies regulate the use of GMOs: the U.S. Food and Drug Administration, the U.S. Environmental Protection Agency (EPA), and the U.S. Department of Agriculture (USDA). These agencies claim GMOs are safe for consumption, but are they really? These organizations are the same ones that refuse to ban ingredients that other countries have banned because of their significant health concerns. I, for one, don't fully trust them to make sure what I am eating is actually safe. Also, how can they really know? When we are only a few decades into GMO consumption, it's not possible to be certain they pose no long-term health risks.

Some evidence, in fact, has suggested they do![32] That's why there are more than 60 countries worldwide that require companies to label GMO products. If you'd like to learn more about which countries require labeling (and which ones do not), check out the Center for Food Safety website that is listed at the end of this book.[33] You might have heard of the National Bioengineered Food Disclosure Standard (NBFDS). In 2018, Congress passed a law requiring some labeling of genetically modified organisms. *Some* labeling. Not all.

As of 2022, many products containing GMOs include labels reading "Bioengineered" or something similar. Unfortunately, there are many exemptions to this law, including meat from animals that have been fed GMO feed and food sold in restaurants. Restaurants can use GMOs without having to tell the consumer in any way.

The Non-GMO Project said this about the new law: "In its current form, categorical exemptions prevent this law from delivering the meaningful protections Americans deserve. Highly processed ingredients ... and many meat and dairy products will not require disclosure. Animal feed is not covered by this law; meat, eggs, and dairy from animals fed a GMO diet will not require a disclosure. Overall, many products containing GMOs will not be labeled, meaning that the absence of a bioengineered (BE) disclosure does not mean a product is non-GMO."[34]

Though this law is definitely a step in the right direction, it's not good enough. Consumers should know what they are eating at all times. They shouldn't have to guess or read between the lines. Labels should be clear 100 percent of the time.

In the United States, the following crops are often genetically modified:[35]

- Corn
- Soybeans
- Cotton
- Sugar beets
- Alfalfa
- Apples
- Canola
- Potatoes
- Eggplants
- Papayas
- Pineapples
- Salmon
- Squash

Many people look at a short list like this and think, *Not too bad. As long as I avoid these specific crops, I should be fine, right?* Sadly, no. These products find their way into many—dare I say MOST—of the food we eat in the United States.

According to the FDA, "In 2018, GMO soybeans made up 94% of all soybeans planted, GMO cotton made up 94% of all cotton planted, and 92% of corn planted was GMO corn."[36] It's the same story with canola and sugar beets. If you are eating anything that contains soy, corn, canola, cotton, or sugar beets (this includes granulated sugar), you are VERY likely consuming a genetically modified crop.

What's worse, many of these GMO plants are used to make other ingredients that are often used in packaged foods. Look for ingredients like cornstarch, corn syrup, granulated sugar, soybean oil, corn oil, soy lecithin, cottonseed oil, hydrolyzed vegetable protein, and sweeteners. Consumers can't avoid GMOs by avoiding GMO produce alone. They have to also avoid any product made with the produce, and here in the United States that is quite a large number of products! GMOs are hidden in our food supply in massive amounts. In particular, they like to linger in processed foods. Restaurants, likewise, are GMO minefields, unless, of course, they serve organic produce and animal products. Most, in my experience, do not.

So, what's the big deal? Why does this even matter? While there is a lack of credible human studies on the health effects of GMOs, there is plenty of evidence to recognize many of the risks associated with regular consumption of these lab-derived food-like substances.

As mentioned earlier, one of the primary causes of concern with GMOs is the increase of herbicide usage. There is research that suggests that the increase of GMOs, resulting in the increase of herbicides, can be detrimental to our health. Some of those health concerns include the following: gastrointestinal disorders, obesity, diabetes, heart disease, depression, autism, infertility, cancer, Alzheimer's disease, kidney disease, osteoporosis, cancer, infertility, neurological disorders (such as ADHD), and others.[37]

The truth is, there are no long-term studies showing the safety of genetically modified organisms. Since they haven't been in our food supply for very long, we don't know what damage they might be doing to us long-term. What we do know, however, is that many diseases have been on the rise since their introduction.

Since the early 1990s (when GMOs really hit the market), Americans have grown sicker and sicker.[38] Food allergies, autism, reproductive issues, cancers, diabetes, heart conditions, and digestive conditions like Crohn's disease, ulcerative colitis, inflammatory bowel disease, and so on have all become more common. Health concerns are rising. Now, admittedly, there are likely several factors involved in the increase of diseases in our country, but GMOs are likely playing a role as well.

When we consume GMOs, we are participating in the ONLY long-term safety trial EVER conducted on humans. I don't know about you, but I don't like the idea of participating in this study, and I most definitely don't like the idea of signing my children up to participate in it either.

Nonetheless, every time I grab a nonorganic product that contains corn, soy, or one of the other plants previously listed, I am doing just that. We don't know how safe or how dangerous GMOs are. I, for one, would rather not take the risk.

Not only are GMOs potentially dangerous for human consumption, but they also pose risks for animals, for farmers, and for the environment. In 2009, the American Academy of Environmental Medicine said, "Several animal studies indicate serious health risks associated with GM food consumption."[39] These risks include immune system disorders, accelerated aging, infertility, and notable changes in certain major organs and the gastrointestinal system.

More than 95 percent of the animals used for meat and dairy in the United States eat food that has been genetically modified.[40] The FDA reassures us that even though our animals eat GMOs, the DNA from the food doesn't make it into our food supply. But again, do you trust their word? I don't. How are we injuring our animals by stuffing them full of GMOs? How are we injuring ourselves?

Though there are certainly positive aspects of GMOs for farmers such as those noted previously, there are also risks. "Because GMOs are novel life forms, biotechnology companies have been able to obtain patents to control the use and distribution of their genetically engineered seeds. Genetically modified crops therefore pose a serious threat to farmer sovereignty and to the national food security of any country where they are grown."[41] One of the key tenets of living and working in the United States is the freedom to choose. The widespread use of GMOs in this country is taking away that freedom from many of our hard-working farmers.

As stated, the majority of genetically modified crops in the United States (up to 80 percent) are made to withstand herbicide application.[42] Because of this, farmers are using significantly larger amounts of herbicides to kill weeds on their land. The chemicals in these herbicides, in particular glyphosate, are potentially carcinogenic to humans—which alone is bad enough—but these chemicals are also creating superweeds. Superweeds are able to survive typical herbicides and are only killed by even stronger chemicals.

I can only imagine what's coming next if our country continues to rely on GMOs for the majority of the food supply. Are these superweeds going to continue to adapt and become stronger as well? Are farmers going to have to continue spraying with even stronger (and more dangerous) chemicals as time goes on? It would certainly seem that way—UNLESS something changes.

One of my favorite movie scenes is from the 2012 children's movie *The Lorax*, which is based on the 1971 book by Dr. Seuss. In this movie, the Lorax is the protector of the trees. Throughout the movie, he is trying to stop the Once-ler from destroying the gorgeous trees of Thneedville. But the Once-ler won't listen to the Lorax. He needs the leaves on the trees to create products for his thriving business. It's possible for him to pluck the leaves instead of bulldozing the trees, but the Once-ler doesn't want to wait. He wants results, and he wants them fast.

Eventually, because of his ever-growing desire for more, he ends up killing all of the trees in the town. The entire city becomes treeless, so much so that they have to manufacture air.

Years later, a young boy in the city named Ted has heard stories about trees and wants to plant one. Only one seed remains, legends say, and it belongs to the Once-ler, who lives outside of town. When Ted finds the Once-ler's broken-down home, the Once-ler shares a lesson he learned the hard way: "Unless someone like you cares a whole awful lot, nothing is going to get better. It's not." The Once-ler gives Ted the remaining tree seed and encourages him to be the difference.

> "UNLESS SOMEONE LIKE YOU CARES A WHOLE AWFUL LOT, NOTHING IS GOING TO GET BETTER. IT'S NOT."
> – DR. SEUSS

It's an animated movie. A fictional tale. But, like many of Dr. Seuss's works, it contains a valuable lesson for us. Nothing is ever going to change unless we care enough to do something about it. Do you want fewer GMOs in our food supply? Do you care enough about the health of your family to live differently, to shop differently, to spend your money differently? In the pages ahead, I'm going to share a few things we can all do to make a difference. To be the difference.

What Can One Person Do?

I used to think I was powerless to make any kind of difference. After all, we're talking about the United States government here. We're talking about changing the food supply of an entire nation. I'm not a scientist or a politician. Heck, I'm not even originally from this country. I'm an Aussie, living here in the United States with my family, running a business, raising my children and, sometimes, just trying to make it through the day. What can one person do?

I think that's the wrong question to ask, though. It's not about what one person can do. It's about the ripple effect. What you or I do might not make a global difference today. But if we change our families and impact our small sectors of the world and then our families continue to do the same, the ripple effect can eventually become massive. Like a tsunami that grows larger and larger as it moves through the ocean and nears land, so also can our impact grow to mammoth proportions as it spreads outside of our family unit.

What can we do? The first step—and most important step—in changing the GMO industry is to buy organic non-GMO foods when possible. One of the most common questions caregivers ask when beginning to eat healthier is this: "Do we really need to buy organic? It's so much more expensive." I can certainly relate to this challenge, as organic produce IS more expensive than nonorganic. In some cases, it's not necessary to buy organic because, as you now know, not all crops are genetically modified and some are less likely to be contaminated with pesticides or other toxic chemicals. But in other cases, it is the single most important thing you can do to protect your family from the dangers of genetically modified organisms and other toxins.

What I suggest to families I work with is to check out the Environmental Working Group (EWG) website. Each year, the EWG puts out updated Dirty Dozen and Clean 15 lists, detailing which foods are the "dirtiest" (meaning they have the most pesticides) and which foods are the "cleanest." In 2022, the foods on the dirty dozen list included the following: strawberries, spinach, kale, collard, mustard greens, nectarines, apples, grapes, cherries, peaches, pears, bell and hot peppers, celery, and tomatoes. When seeking to eat clean produce, stick with organic for these foods, as well as for corn, papaya, and summer squash, since these foods are very heavily genetically modified in the United States.

This is the greatest thing you can do for yourself and for your family to stop ingesting toxic chemicals and mystery organisms. It's also the greatest thing you can personally do to effect change. Money talks, and if enough of us stop buying certain products, companies will eventually stop producing them. Change only happens when people care enough to do something about it. If we want the food industry to care enough, we have to speak in their language—and that language is the dollar bill. Buy organic and non-GMO when finances allow. This single change is the MOST beneficial thing you can do to protect your family from the inherent risks of GMOs.

You might be curious what it means for a product to be certified organic. In essence, it means that these products are grown or raised on farms that do NOT use any prohibited substances, such as most synthetic fertilizers and pesticides, sewage sludge, or genetic engineering. Organic farmers use only natural processes on their farms, so when we buy organic, we can know for sure that we are not eating GMOs or toxic chemicals. For more information about what makes a product organic, check out the fact sheet from the USDA in the notes at the end of this book. It describes in detail the practices organic farmers must use to prevent pests and weeds, rotate crops, and raise and feed livestock.[43]

Many of the families I work with find that shopping at their local farmers' markets helps them find clean fruits and vegetables. By shopping locally, families can speak directly with the farmers. Sometimes, farmers might not be certified organic (as that can be expensive for a farmer) but might still follow organic practices. Get to know the farmers in your area, and you might find many who follow organic practices, even if they don't have the organic label.

A second step we can take to effect change is to eliminate processed foods from our diet. Most of them contain GMOs, as we've already discussed, so cutting them out completely will eliminate a large portion of GMOs from your diet. Of course, it might not be realistic to cut out processed foods 100 percent. For many busy families like my own—and especially those of us with kids—cutting out processed foods entirely takes far too much time in the kitchen. If you're like my family—often busy and not wanting to make everything from scratch—then buy products that are labeled non-GMO. These products are the future of the anti-GMO movement. The more support non-GMO products can get, the higher the demand for them will be.

I wonder what would happen if people refused to buy GMO products and exclusively bought foods labeled non-GMO? If profits plummeted, do you think companies would make some changes? I'm certain they would! We aren't powerless in this. Because we hold the cash, we hold the power. If a company can boost sales significantly by creating a non-GMO product, they will find a way to make it happen. We just need to convince them there's a market for non-GMO products!

Third, push for GMO labeling. I think everyone can agree, it's our right to know exactly what we're putting into our bodies. If a company is using GMO ingredients, fine. That's its prerogative. But it should be required to tell us. The United States has taken steps in the right direction with the National Bioengineered Food Disclosure Standard, but because of the many exceptions included in this law, it's not good enough. We still don't clearly know what's in our food supply. One way we can do this is to reach out to our local lawmakers and congress members, asking them to create laws that require better GMO labeling.

In *The Lorax,* Ted was the one who cared enough to make a difference. He was the one who planted that seed and brought trees (and breathable air!) back into the town of Thneedville. You and I have the chance to do the same thing today in our cities. We have the chance to change the health of our families, the freedom of our farmers, the well-being of our animals, and the state of our environment. Will you join me in creating this ripple effect?

What About Meat?

In this chapter, we've talked a lot about produce and the importance of buying clean produce that has not been genetically modified and that has not been smothered with chemicals. But what about meat? Is it important to buy organic meat too? This is a great question, and the answer is YES!

If your budget allows you to buy organic, grass-fed or wild-caught protein sources, that is the best way to go. The organic seal on meat means the animals were raised on land that hasn't been subjected to any prohibited substances for at least three years. That means no pesticides, fertilizers, or other potentially dangerous substances. It also means the animals had access to the outdoors year-round—at all times. They were fed an organic diet and not given antibiotics or hormones. To be considered fully grass-fed, the animal has to eat only grass for its entire life, as soon as it is weaned from its mother's milk. Make sure when buying beef that it is also grass-finished. Some cattle are raised on grass but then finished at a feedlot with grain to fatten them up. The ideal is to have grass-fed and grass-finished organic beef. It is possible to be grass-fed but NOT organic. For this reason, it's best to look for both grass-fed AND organic.

As far as fish is concerned, it's best to purchase wild-caught fish. Wild-caught fish are raised in their natural environment and eat a variety of krill and other tiny shellfish. In contrast, farm-raised fish are often raised in a large tank and can be fed fish feed that contains artificial ingredients. What our food eats, we eat. That's why it's so important to choose the highest quality protein sources. Wild-caught fish are also typically higher in essential minerals and lower in saturated fat than farm-raised fish, making them a much healthier option.

Chapter Highlights

- GMO stands for "genetically modified organism."
- GMOs are created using four steps: 1) identify the appealing gene in the original organism, 2) copy the information from that gene, 3) insert that genetic information into another organism, and 4) grow a new organism.
- In the United States, the following crops are often genetically modified: corn, soybeans, cotton, sugar beets, alfalfa, apples, canola, potatoes, eggplant, papaya, pineapple, salmon, and squash.
- Pros of GMOs: When using GMOs, farmers are able to produce more plants with fewer resources. There are fewer crops destroyed by insects or weeds. GMOs also reduce insecticide use.

- Cons of GMOs: Herbicide usage has gone up since the introduction of GMOs, leading to an increase in glyphosate contamination in our food supply. GMOs are potentially linked to health concerns in both humans and animals. They are also creating "superweeds" that require even stronger chemicals to kill. Because GMOs are patented, farmers are losing some of their rights. There are no long-term health studies proving the safety of consuming GMOs. (We are participating in the ONLY long-term study every time we eat them.)

- Even though the United States has taken some steps in the right direction as far as labeling GMO products goes, there is still much work to be done! ALL products containing GMOs should be labeled—not just some of them.

- We CAN make a difference! Remember the wise advice from our friend Dr. Seuss: "Unless someone like you cares a whole awful lot, nothing is going to get better. It's not."

- When finances allow, buy organic and non-GMO foods.

- When purchasing meat, stick with grass-fed, organic, and wild-caught if possible.

Action Steps

1. Read *The Lorax* by Dr. Seuss with your family this week, and then watch the movie by the same name. Use these as a springboard to talk about some of the changes you plan to make, moving forward.

2. Look at the current EWG (Environmental Working Group) Dirty Dozen and Clean 15 lists. Better yet, download a copy of the Dirty Dozen list from their website if it's available. A new list typically comes out each year. Stick this list in your car or purse and use it every time you shop for produce. Buy organic produce if the food item is on the Dirty Dozen list.

3. What are five processed foods you can eliminate from your diet? Think of five products you want to get rid of and the foods you can eat instead to replace these items. (For instance, could you cut out chips from your diet and save them for rare occasions only? You could replace chips with homemade trail mix or with fruit and nut butter.)

4. Consider reaching out to your local lawmakers and congress members, asking them to create laws that require better GMO labeling.

CHAPTER 6:
Meal Planning 101

There's an old saying attributed to Benjamin Franklin that reads, "If you fail to plan, you plan to fail." That is definitely true in natural ADHD symptom reduction! Caregivers who don't plan their family's meals will likely end up eating out or popping a frozen pizza into the oven. That was definitely my default before I began meal planning.

It's also what happened with Shayla and her husband, Eric. Shayla and Eric both have full-time jobs outside the home. They are both teachers, so they also live on a limited income. They learned on their own about the damaging effects of gluten and dairy and how these two foods in particular can aggravate ADHD symptoms. They have two kids with ADHD, Katie and Josh. Katie is seven and Josh is twelve.

Before I met their family, Shayla and Eric had already cut both dairy and gluten entirely from their family's diet. Well ... not entirely. When Shayla and I chatted on the phone after she joined our program, she said that about once a week, usually on a Thursday evening, they ended up ordering takeout. Both of their kids refused healthier options when they went out and often ended up eating something with either gluten or dairy or both in it.

"Honestly, I just don't have the energy to fight them on it. It's not worth it," she told me on the phone.

Something she said, though, struck a nerve with me: "... usually on a Thursday." It made me wonder if that day of the week was the key to figuring out their lack of progress.

"Why do you think it's usually a Thursday that you go out to eat?" I asked her.

"Both my husband and I are usually really tired by Thursday. We just don't want to cook. And the thought of having to figure out something healthy to eat feels too big when I'm already so tired from work."

"That makes sense," I reassured her. "But I don't think the problem actually starts on Thursday. I think it starts the weekend before."

As we talked more about how their family functioned, I learned that their weeks are usually extremely busy. Katie, their seven-year-old, takes dance classes several times a week. Josh, their twelve-year-old, has football practice every night during the fall, basketball in the winter, and soccer in the spring. They're also involved with their local church, and in the evenings they have to grade papers and prepare lesson plans. It's no wonder they're exhausted by Thursday night each week!

"This dietary change is never going to give you the results you want to see if you don't start doing something differently BEFORE Thursday hits," I told her. Then we talked about the importance of meal planning. "The whole purpose of meal planning is so that you cook more meals at once and then limit the amount of time you have to spend in the kitchen later on. You shouldn't be cooking on Thursday nights if you're always tired. You should be cooking your Thursday meal the weekend before, so Thursdays are work- and stress-free."

In the pages ahead, I'm going to teach you how to plan meals using the same steps I taught Shayla. I used to think of meal planning as a necessary drudgery—something I hated doing but definitely needed to do. By the end of this chapter, you might view it like that too: a necessary drudgery. My hope, though, is that you'll learn enough tips and tricks that meal planning will no longer be such a drag.

Why Plan Meals?

Before we dive into the how-to of meal planning, let's explore WHY it's so critical. When we understand WHY we do something, it can help us stick with it when the going gets tough. I'll admit that meal planning is not my favorite "adulting" activity. It's actually one of the things I would prefer not to do. But I do it each week because I understand the benefits so clearly.

First of all, meal planning and prepping saves time throughout the busy workweek. Granted, it does take more time on the front end than many people are used to spending. But the time they spend on the front end saves them HOURS throughout the week. It's not so much the amount of time as the allocation of time. Instead of working on meals each night when you're already tired from a long workday, meal planning allows you to do most of the work on the weekend so that time is freed up during the week. Most busy families find this to be the number one reason they choose to plan and prep meals on the weekends.

A second benefit of meal planning is that it saves money. Unfortunately, eating healthy is more expensive than eating SAD (aka the Standard American Diet). Because healthier foods are more expensive, many families are looking for ways to save money. Meal planning is one of the primary tools they can use to accomplish this goal. Why? Because when we plan meals, we are less likely to order takeout. The markup for takeout is mammoth, so most families find they end up saving money when they plan meals because they eat out less often.

One mom told me recently, "I thought we would be spending tons more on food because we are eating this way. And even though our grocery bill has definitely gone up, our overall spending on food has actually gone down because we don't eat out as often. I was shocked by how much money we were throwing away on takeout!"

What this mom learned is that it's significantly cheaper to eat at home than to eat at a restaurant—even when eating organic food! We can eat a steak at home for about half the price of a steak at a restaurant. Likewise for hamburgers or chicken strips. We can feed a family of four for about half as much money if we feed them at home than if we feed them at a restaurant (and in some cases there's an even greater price difference)!

Meal planning also saves us money because it allows us to buy in bulk and to have a better idea of the staples we need to have on hand. That way, when one of these staples goes on sale, we can grab several of them, knowing they will not go to waste. Nearly every product is priced better in bulk. Meal planners can use this information to their advantage by planning meals with products they can purchase in bulk.

Planning meals also saves us money because meal planners typically shop for groceries with a list. Remember, the food industry has marketing down to a science. They know how to get people to buy something. If shoppers go to the store without a list, they are MUCH more likely to buy something they don't need. Shopping with a list prevents those impulse buys.

My children love the Marvel movies. Have you seen them? *Iron Man, Captain America* (my favorite superhero), *Spider-Man, Ant-Man*, and the rest? Think of your shopping list like Tony Stark's Iron Man suit. When Tony wears the suit, no weapon is getting through it. He's invincible. Your shopping list is like his suit. It blocks the marketing attacks that are aimed at you and keeps those impulse buys from making their way through to you.

A third benefit of meal planning is that you will become healthier by default. Just by eating at home more often, you will cut down on calories, additives, and processed foods! By meal planning, you have full control over what your family eats. Instead of being dictated by your hunger pangs, you will follow the plan laid out earlier in the week.

Kelly was a petite woman. If I had to guess, I would imagine she didn't weigh more than 120 pounds when her family joined my program to help her 8-year-old son, Casen. By looking at her, I would never have guessed she had high cholesterol. But she did. Kelly told me later that she was 19 years old and 105 pounds when she first learned she had cholesterol issues. Kelly's total cholesterol was 200 at that time—not considered high just yet but right on the line. It was what the medical community called "borderline high." It hovered right around 200 throughout Kelly's 20s. Then, as she hit 30, it started to slowly creep up. She was 35 years old when they joined my program and changed the way her family ate.

Kelly's cholesterol dropped from 229 to 187 in one year, just by changing her diet. "It really was meal planning that made the difference for me," she told me. "Meal planning kept us from ordering takeout." Most of our children don't need to worry about cholesterol and weight, but some of us adults might. Many of the families I work with have been surprised at how their own health improved because of the changes they made for their children.

Heather saw the same thing as Kelly. Her cholesterol dropped 30 points because of the dietary changes she made.

Heather
6 hrs

Good morning guys! I had forgotten to mention this during our group coaching call which I'm sure you noticed I dropped off because my battery always seems to tank during those video calls. I apologize! I have been following the gluten free dairy free diet along with my family for 2 months now. I had my yearly physical and my cholesterol dropped 30 points which put me in a normal range for the 1st time since I can remember. And my thyroid function increased. I don't know if it's from this change, but my doctor was very happy when I had my results!

Amy, like both Heather and Kelly, also saw health improvements. She had battled chronic hip pain for years and was ready to try medication to get some relief. But then she joined our program to help her child with his ADHD, and guess what? Her pain went away completely!

Amy : I'll share! We started the program in March. We are hoping to start her next level of testing soon (which many start with at the beginning), as we can tell something else needs to be eliminated. We've noticed a lot less anxiety, improved speech, much more calmness, and better ability to focus in our child. His not as moody, more in control of his emotions, able to share what he is feeling, and generally not as 'loud' all day long. I've finally been able to have real discussions and two way conversations with him, that he wasn't really capable of before. Our entire family follows the program. I personally have benefited from the changes. I had some chronic pain that I've lived with for years. I was actually in the process of discussing with my doctor for further evaluation and possible medication for. Once we started some dietary eliminations, the pain completely went away! Several foods were causing me inflammation. I feel so much younger now that I can move again. It made me realize just how much certain foods could be impacting our kid's system. Feel free to PM me if you have questions.

Like · Reply · 20h · Edited

What so many of our caregivers find when working to reduce their children's ADHD symptoms naturally is that the inflammation in their own bodies improves as well. Inflammation in the body isn't just something our children deal with! It's something we all experience when we eat foods like gluten, dairy, and soy. But just think: if we as adults—who have likely been eating poorly for many years—can have such quick and amazing results, what might happen with our children? How quickly might you see results in them? Meal planning can help you get to those results faster!

A fourth meal-planning benefit is that it can prevent food waste. When families plan meals, they have a better idea of the foods that are in their fridge. They only buy food they are going to eat, and they stick to their plan, thus keeping waste to a minimum.

Think back to Shayla and Eric. Why did they order takeout every Thursday night? Was it because they wanted to eat that? Or was it because it was easy and convenient? If you thought, "easy and convenient," you're 100 percent correct. Many times, we aren't addicted to junk food because of the food; we're addicted to junk food because of the convenience. Meal planning makes healthy food easy and convenient.

> WE AREN'T ADDICTED TO JUNK FOOD BECAUSE OF THE FOOD; WE'RE ADDICTED TO JUNK FOOD BECAUSE OF CONVENIENCE.

Meal Planning Steps

Meal planning isn't hard, but there are a few critical steps that will help you be successful. We'll walk through each of these steps now in detail.

Step 1: Review the Calendar

The first step is to take a look at your calendar for the upcoming week. What events do you have going on? Are there any scheduled meals out or with friends or family? Are there nights when you anticipate you will be tired and not want to cook? Do you have any events that occur during the dinner hour? Jot any of these activities down on a notepad or calendar.

Step 2: Choose Meals

The second step, once you have looked at your calendar, is to choose meals for each day of the upcoming week: breakfast, lunch, dinner, and snacks. I recommend planning all of your meals and snacks for each day, but if this feels like too much to begin with, choose one per day and start there. You can always work your way up to more later on when you feel ready. I also recommend choosing some meals that require more time and some that are quicker, just in case plans change throughout the week, so that you have flexibility to swap out a couple of meals to accommodate the change.

To make this step easier moving forward, create four running lists of your family's favorite gluten-free/dairy-free/soy-free meals: one list for breakfast, one list for lunch, one list for dinner, and one list for snacks. As you find a meal that your family enjoys, add it to the list. Soon, you'll have a surplus of meals and snack ideas to choose from to help you with meal planning. We have even created a template to help make this easy for you. Scan this QR code to get a free copy of our printable Family Favorite Meal List Template.

Step 3: Plug the Meals into Your Calendar

Now that you have chosen your meals and reviewed your calendar, the next step is to plug the meals into your calendar where you think they will work best. Remember, if you know you're going to be tired and not wanting to cook one evening, plan a quick meal for that night or plan something that you can fully prepare ahead of time.

Step 4: Make a Grocery List, and Then Shop for Items on the List

Step 4 is to make a grocery list and shop for the ingredients you need. Looking at each meal on your meal plan, write down any ingredients you need to purchase. Make sure you are thinking through snacks as you make your list too. There's nothing more frustrating than returning from the grocery store and realizing you forgot some of the items you will need for the week. When you go to the store, only buy items that are on the list. THIS is where meal planning starts to save you money! If it's not on the list, it doesn't go in the cart.

> IF IT'S NOT ON THE LIST, IT DOESN'T GO IN THE CART.

Step 5: Prepare What You Can Ahead of Time

Step 5 is to think through what can be prepared ahead of time. Can you chop veggies? Can you cut fruit? Can you thaw or cook your meat? Can you mix ingredients? Choose a window of time on the weekend that would be good for you to prepare your meals. Do as much as you can during this window of time. Wash and cut fruit and vegetables that you will eat throughout the week. Cook meat for the next few days if your chosen recipes allow precooking. Mix ingredients. As you first get started, this can feel like a lot of work, but the relaxation it provides during the hectic workweek is worth it 100 percent.

Step 6: Label and Store Prepared Ingredients

The final step in the process, once you have chosen your meals, written them all down, shopped, and prepped, is to label and store the ingredients in your fridge so that you know exactly where everything is and when you need to use it.

Tips from Those in the Trenches

I asked the families in my program to share some of their best tips and tricks that make meal planning easier for them. Here are some of their responses and my additional suggestions:

Cathy: "Give yourself plenty of time to plan meals and prep, especially when you're first starting out." My recommendation is to allot an hour or two each week for Steps 1–4 when you first start meal planning. Allot another hour or two to prep meals. I know two to four hours on a weekend sounds like a lot (and it is!), but that means you have two to four fewer hours each week that you have to be in the kitchen. The trade-off has been beneficial for all of the families I work with.

Tim: "Scan your fridge or pantry for items that need to be eaten soon and incorporate them into your family's meal plan." This is excellent advice and can save some families a significant amount of money. It also creates less food waste because the food you already have is eaten, rather than tossed in the trash a few days later, after it has gone bad.

Alex: "Meal planning doesn't mean everything has to be homemade!" This might be my favorite piece of advice because many families assume meal planning means you never get to go out to eat. That's not the case! It's okay to plan for takeout. Just put that on the meal plan beforehand. One benefit of adding this to your meal plan beforehand is that you can research the restaurant ahead of time and know exactly what gluten-free, dairy-free options they serve. Many restaurants have allergen menus online that you can find. If that's not available at the restaurant you plan to patronize, then you can call and ask to speak to the manager ahead of time. Another great tool is the Find Me Gluten Free app. This app provides information about local gluten-free restaurants and options near you.

Renee: "I love to pre-make my smoothies. This has helped us in the morning big time as we try to get out the door for school." For smoothies, put all the ingredients except the liquids in a labeled bag or container and pop it into the fridge or freezer for later use. Add the liquid and the bagged ingredients to your blender when you are ready to mix. Enjoy.

Andrea: "Have a backup plan in your freezer at all times." There are going to be meals that totally flop. There are going to be times when you are too tired to cook what you had planned. These backup meals are lifesavers! One of my personal favorites is gluten-free, precooked breakfast sausages with a side of fruit or oven fries.

Val: "Double up on dinners so you have leftovers as a meal the next day." This is my favorite way to plan for lunch. We double the dinner recipe and plan for my kids to take the leftovers to school the next day for lunch. Alternatively, you could double up your recipes so that you have enough for a second dinner.

Meal planning was the key to Shayla and Eric's challenges with gluten-free and dairy-free eating. Once they started meal planning, they were able to finally become 100 percent gluten- and dairy-free. THAT was when they started seeing real changes in their children. Meal planning might not ever be your favorite thing to do (it still isn't mine!), but if it leads to better or quicker results, it's worth it 100 percent!

Chapter Highlights

- Meal planning and prepping has the following benefits:
  - It saves time
  - It saves money
  - It keeps families healthier
  - It prevents food waste
- Meal planning can be broken down into the following steps:
  - Review your calendar for the upcoming week
  - Choose meals for each day of the upcoming week (breakfast, lunch, dinner, and snacks)
  - Write down each of your chosen meals onto your calendar or meal planner
  - Make a grocery list and shop for the ingredients you need
  - Prepare as much of the food as you can ahead of time
  - Label and store the prepared food

Action Steps

1. Take an hour or two to plan your meals for the coming week. Think through and list your plans for the following: breakfast, lunch, dinner, morning snack, and afternoon snack. Review the steps covered previously as you plan your meals.

2. Create four running lists of your family's favorite gluten-free/dairy-free/soy-free meals: one list for breakfast, one list for lunch, one list for dinner, and one list for snacks. As you find a meal that your family enjoys, add it to the list. Soon, you'll have a surplus of meals and snack ideas to choose from to help you with meal planning. Want us to do the work for you? Scan this QR code to get a free copy of our printable Family Favorite Meal List Template.

3 Look over the tips from other caregivers. Which one of these do you plan to put into practice? Add a star next to your favorite tips.

CHAPTER 7:

Hidden Sources of Gluten, Dairy, and Soy

Many caregivers of children with ADHD *think* they have removed gluten, dairy, and soy from their children's diets, but later find out there were hidden sources of these foods finding their way into some of their staple products. That's what happened to Kasey and Jack and their daughter, Jennifer.

Kasey and Jack decided they were going to remove gluten, dairy, and soy from their entire family's diet, primarily to help their daughter, Jennifer. Jennifer had ADHD, along with autism spectrum disorder (ASD) and oppositional defiant disorder (ODD).

When Kasey and Jack first contacted me, we decided to do functional lab testing for them because of some significant symptoms Jennifer was experiencing. She not only had the classic ADHD, ASD, and ODD symptoms but also some gut problems such as constipation, upset stomach, bloating, and gas.

After completing the tests, we saw A LOT of underlying stressors in Jennifer's body. She had a couple of parasites but also an overgrowth of bacteria in her gut, as well as *Helicobacter pylori* and *candida*. If you don't know what these words mean, that's totally okay. Suffice it to say, she had a significant amount of distress in her body—so much so that I knew we would probably not be able to target it all in only one round of supplementation. I knew we would probably need to do a second round of testing, followed by a second round of supplements as well. There are some occasions when there is so much going on in the body that a second round of targeted supplementation is necessary, and this was one of those occasions.

When Kasey and Jack saw Jennifer's test results, they took swift action and removed gluten, dairy, and soy immediately from their pantry and refrigerator. Jennifer's body was reacting strongly to gluten, so they didn't want it in the house at all. They assumed that if it was in the house, she would sneak it, so they removed that temptation. They also removed the 14 other foods Jennifer was sensitive to.

About six months later, they had worked through the first round of targeted supplementation. We wanted to see how Jennifer's gut had improved, so we ran a second round of tests. When we got the results back, I saw something that concerned me: significant gluten exposure. Her tests made it abundantly clear that Jennifer was not, in fact, as gluten-free as her parents had assumed. The test results of a gluten-free individual look significantly different than the test results of someone who is eating gluten, and hers were definitely the results of someone eating gluten.

When I shared these results with Kasey and Jack, they were baffled. "I really don't understand," Kasey told me. "We don't have gluten in the house. She's hardly ever with anyone besides us. We even homeschool, so I don't know where she could be getting it."

I was writing this chapter right about that same time, so I sent it to her to read through. "I want you to look through this chapter and see if there could be some hidden sources of gluten in your house," I told her.

A week later, she texted me. "I had no idea gluten could be in lunchmeat. Jennifer was eating lunchmeat at least twice a week, and the brand we have been using has gluten in it!" Kasey was a diligent label-reader for most foods but had neglected to look at her family's lunchmeat. She assumed there wouldn't be gluten in there because, really, why would there be gluten in meat?

Even after being on this journey for years, I am still shocked by how many foods contain gluten. I picked up a bag of frozen carrots and peas at the store the other day and saw the warning, "May contain gluten." In carrots and peas! Why in the world would a frozen vegetable possibly contain gluten? It was a reminder to me that I have to stay diligent. Just because a food *shouldn't* have gluten in it does not mean a food *doesn't* have gluten in it.

It's also important to continue to read the labels on packaged foods that have previously been free of gluten. Sometimes, companies change their recipes and introduce gluten into a previously gluten-free product. One of my clients showed me two bags of chips that were a staple product in her home: one she had purchased a few weeks prior and one she purchased that day. One of them had gluten in it; the other did not. The recipe had changed. Unfortunately, you cannot assume that just because a product was gluten-free in the past, it will remain gluten-free forever. It's critical to continue reading labels diligently.

> **JUST BECAUSE A FOOD *SHOULDN'T* HAVE GLUTEN IN IT DOES NOT MEAN IT *DOESN'T* HAVE GLUTEN IN IT.**

In the pages ahead, I'm going to walk through some of the most common sources of hidden gluten, dairy, and soy. As you read through this chapter, feel free to plug in a bookmark and run to your pantry to check those labels!

Meat, Fish, and Poultry

Many families, like Kasey and Jack's, assume that meat, fish, and poultry are safe. These foods aren't ones most people typically think of when they think of gluten, but unfortunately they sometimes contain gluten, especially the processed varieties like deli meat, hot dogs, and salami. Look out for the words "hydrolyzed wheat protein" in these types of products. If you like to buy chicken that has already been seasoned, you'll also need to be careful, as many seasonings have gluten added as well. Meat and fish substitutes, like veggie burgers, for instance, also often contain gluten.

Potato Chips and Fries

Potatoes are naturally gluten-free, so chips and fries should be safe, right? In theory, yes, but definitely not in practice. Many chips and french fries are coated in gluten before they are cooked.

When we first began this journey, french fries were the hidden source of gluten for us. It was several months after removing gluten that I learned that many fries served in restaurants are coated in gluten before they are cooked. It's important to check restaurant menus for allergens BEFORE ordering so that you're aware of the ingredients that are added to their products.

Another issue with french fries and potato chips, especially those served at restaurants, is that they are often fried in the same oil as gluten products. For instance, the fries at a restaurant might be fried in the same oil as chicken strips that are covered with gluten.

Every family is different as far as cross-contamination is concerned. Some children have such a strong response to gluten that it is critical for them to avoid cross-contamination like that from using a shared grill or frier. For other families, though, as long as it is not direct ingestion of gluten, cross-contamination is not something to stress over. Without testing, it's impossible to know exactly how reactive a child might be to gluten.

What I typically recommend to families who are not testing is to avoid direct ingestion of gluten. If after three to six months they still are not seeing the improvement they would like to see, they can then begin avoiding cross-contamination as well.

Another strategy to help with cross-contamination is to take a digestive enzyme supplement that is specifically designed to help with the digestion of wheat when you are eating out at a restaurant. Sadly, many times families have told me horror stories of requesting gluten-free items at a restaurant and then still experiencing gluten reactions afterward. I have learned the hard way that many restaurants serving gluten-free foods still have significant cross-contamination. When my family eats out, we all take a digestive enzyme before the meal and often take it for a couple meals thereafter as well. If you'd like to know my favorite brand, scan this QR code to get access to my resource page.

Oats

I don't always insist families buy certified gluten-free products. They're expensive and can be unnecessary in many instances. Oats, though, are the exception to this. Oats need to be certified gluten-free to guarantee that they are not contaminated with gluten. That's because oats are one of the most commonly gluten-contaminated foods.

Beverages

Many flavored coffees and teas contain gluten, dairy, or soy. Even when ordering dairy-free milks in coffees and teas, some of the syrups aren't safe and will lead to accidental exposure. Again, the key here is to double-check restaurant menus and labels on products before consuming them.

Eggs

Yep, you read that right. Even eggs can be problematic at restaurants. Eggs by themselves are a wonderful source of protein. In fact, they are a superfood that we discussed in more depth in Chapter 4. But sometimes milk, butter, cheese, sour cream, or even pancake batter is added to eggs before they are cooked.

Always verify with your server at a restaurant that the eggs are gluten- and dairy-free before consuming them. I have found that it's best to tell your server upon arrival that you have a gluten and dairy allergy. They will often note this on your ticket when they submit it to the chef. Then, when our food arrives, I double-check with them that our foods are, in fact, gluten- and dairy-free.

Treats

Some families get caught off guard by the gluten that is sometimes in ice cream. Because they associate ice cream with dairy, they purchase dairy-free ice cream and assume they are safe. Unfortunately, many dairy-free ice creams still contain gluten. For instance, brownie batter or cookie dough dairy-free ice creams, though dairy-free, are usually NOT gluten-free.

Gelato can also be tricky. Some gelato varieties are dairy-free. Others, though, are not. Always read those labels before purchasing or consuming a product. And remember, manufacturing processes change frequently, so don't assume that just because an item was safe in the past that it is still safe today.

Another product that often surprises families is candy. Licorice, in particular, often contains gluten. Milk is commonly found in candy as well, especially in chocolate candies. Even dark chocolate often contains dairy. The only way to ensure you are eating candy that is gluten-, dairy-, and soy-free is to check the label.

Soy is an especially sneaky ingredient and finds its way into thousands of products that families would not expect. Energy bars and granola bars, for instance, often contain soy. They can also contain gluten. Many families buy into the lie that energy products try to sell us: that they are healthy. In reality, many granola bars are nothing more than a well-disguised piece of candy. They contain tons of sugar, along with gluten, dairy, soy, and other ingredients that are far from healthy.

Sauces, Salad Dressings, Soups, and Gravies

Many salad dressings contain gluten. Although salad can be a healthy option, make sure to order your salads with a safe dressing that does not contain gluten, dairy, or soy, as well as without cheese and croutons.

Other sauces often contain incriminating ingredients too. Gluten is often added to sauces, soups, gravies, and so on as a thickening agent. For many creamy soups, you can be confident that milk is an ingredient. If ordering anything from a restaurant that contains a sauce or gravy, it's best to check the allergen menu for more information, because there's a good chance these sauces are not gluten-, dairy-, and soy-free.

Fried Foods

Some fried foods are safe, but others are not. How can you tell the difference? One clue is if the foods are battered. Foods that are battered (like onion rings, fried okra, fried shrimp, chicken nuggets, etc.) are often coated in flour (which contains gluten) before they are fried. Battered fried foods need to be avoided. Other fried foods, like french fries (assuming they are not coated and not cooked in contaminated oil), are safe to consume.

Soy Sauce

I debated whether to include soy sauce in this chapter. Honestly, soy should be avoided, especially by children with ADHD who already have compromised immune systems. If you need a refresher, look back at the beginning of this book for why soy should be avoided.

Obviously, then, anyone who is avoiding soy will avoid soy sauce. But I know that some people who are reading this might not be ready to remove soy from their diets just yet. They might think, "I'll start with gluten, since it's the top inflammatory food." If this is you, don't worry. Everyone has to take this journey at their own pace. Every step forward is still a step in the right direction! Keep taking those small steps forward.

For that reason, I wanted to note that most soy sauce contains gluten. Though made of soybeans, soy sauce often has wheat added to it. For that reason, even if you don't avoid soy sauce because of the soy, you should avoid it because of the gluten. Or, at the very least, ensure you buy a variety that is certified gluten-free.

Supplements/Medications

Many supplements or medications contain gluten, dairy, or soy. Check the labels of your commonly used medications and see what they contain. Artificial flavors and colors are also very common in medications. Look for gluten-, dairy-, soy-, and food-dye-free versions of the medications you frequently use. Sometimes, for prescription medications, a doctor will specify on the prescription that it be gluten-free. If your doctor is willing to do this, this is a great way to ensure your medication is gluten-free.

Whole Grains

One of my clients told me about her mother-in-law's misunderstanding about gluten. She thought that if a product was labeled "whole grain" that it was free of gluten. This misconception is common. Whole grain is not the same as gluten-free. In fact, many times whole grains DO contain gluten. Be on guard for tricky labeling of products. Companies think that if they label a product as heart-healthy or "whole" that people will believe them. You and I won't fall for it, at least!

Accidental Exposure?

What should you do if you or your child has accidental exposure to gluten, dairy, or soy? As much as we'd like to think we'll never have an exposure, the truth is, that's not reality with most families (possibly all families). In the culture we live in, gluten, dairy, and soy are everywhere, and the likelihood of being 100 percent gluten-, dairy-, and soy-free all of the time with no slip-ups is slim.

Of course, that's the goal, but with children, we need to understand that slip-ups will probably happen. (If you are worried about a child sneaking gluten, dairy, or soy, stay tuned because we're going to dive deep into that common challenge in a later chapter!) At the very least, cross-contamination will occur. So, what should caregivers do when they suspect accidental (or intentional, if a child is being sneaky) exposure?

There are actually several strategies that can help keep the damage to a minimum and get the gluten out of the body quicker. For both gluten and dairy, there are supplements that can help the body digest them more easily. These supplements aren't meant to give someone a free pass to eat as much gluten and dairy as they want (remember, no supplement can fix a terrible diet), but they will help the body digest small amounts that might occur because of cross-contamination or accidental exposure. If you'd like to have a direct link to learn more or purchase these products, scan this QR code. If you'd rather not use one of these products, you could also pick up some activated charcoal to help flush the toxins out of the body.

Along with these supplements, there are other things you can do to help the body as well. Drink lots of water to flush out the body. Take detox baths a couple of times a week. I typically suggest adding 1–2 cups of magnesium salts and 1 cup baking soda to a bath and soaking for about 20 minutes three times a week. Sweating also helps flush the body of toxins, so get outside. Get active and sweat. Jumping on a trampoline, along with making the body sweat, is also very beneficial for detoxification.

Best Practices to Avoid Accidental Exposure

The strategies previously discussed are great when accidental exposure happens, but if we can prevent it from happening in the first place, that's the goal! Here are a few tips to help keep these exposures to a minimum:

1. Read those labels and menus carefully! This is the absolute best strategy for preventing exposure to gluten, dairy, and soy.
2. When eating out, double-check with the server after your food is brought out that your dietary restrictions have been met.
3. "When in doubt, leave it out."[44] If there is an ingredient on a food product that you are not sure about, it's best to skip the product altogether.

4. When at home, prevent cross-contamination. Use a separate toaster for gluten-free bread (if you plan to continue having gluten bread in the house or if you have used the toaster for gluten bread in the past). Don't share butter, nut butters, or jellies that are used on gluten food. Those crumbs can stick around for a long time. Use a separate sponge or washrag for dishes that contain gluten. The best way to ensure your kitchen does not have cross-contamination is to get gluten out of your kitchen. Cross-contamination can't occur if there's no gluten around.

5. Finally, learn the language. Know which ingredients could possibly contain gluten. I love this list of tricky ingredients from the Cleveland Clinic: "… starch, modified food starch, hydrolyzed vegetable protein, hydrolyzed plant protein, textured vegetable protein, dextrin, maltodextrin, glucose syrup, caramel, malt flavoring, malt extract, malt vinegar (distilled vinegar is okay), brown rice syrup."[45] If you see these ingredients on a product that is not certified gluten-free, it's best to avoid that product.

Someday, I would love to see us living in a society where we don't have to be so diligent, where we can read the ingredients on the back of a product and actually know what they are. I'd love to see us living in a society where foods are made of food—not chemicals.

But that's not the world we live in. Yet. Until that day comes and we are able to convince our country to change the way it processes foods, we must be diligent about label and menu reading. Yes, it's a pain sometimes. I don't deny that. But the benefits for this healthy lifestyle far outweigh the inconveniences of checking labels and reading allergen menus.

Chapter Highlights

- Many families think they are fully gluten-, dairy-, and soy-free but are actually not, because of hidden sources of these foods. Some of the most common hidden sources of gluten, dairy, and soy include:
  - Meat, fish, and poultry
  - Potato chips and fries
  - Oats
  - Beverages
  - Eggs
  - Treats
  - Sauces, salad dressings, soups, and gravies
  - Fried foods
  - Soy sauce
  - Supplements/medications
  - Whole grains
- If you or someone in your family is accidentally exposed to gluten, dairy, or soy, there are some strategies you can use to help flush them out of the body quicker:
  - Consider supplements (See Action Step 2 below for some help!)
  - Drink lots of water
  - Sweat a lot
  - Take detox baths three times a week
  - Jump on a trampoline
- Though accidental exposure is certainly possible, there are steps you can take to ensure this happens only rarely:
  - Read labels and menus carefully
  - When you're not sure about an ingredient, skip that product

- Pay special attention to cross-contamination in your kitchen
- Learn about those tricky ingredients that sometimes contain gluten
- Double-check with your server when eating out that they remembered your dietary needs

Action Steps

1. Using the previous list as your guide, look through your pantry and refrigerator for any hidden sources of gluten, dairy, or soy.

2. For accidental exposure to gluten and dairy, there are supplements that can help the body digest them more easily. These supplements aren't meant to give someone a free pass to eat as much gluten and dairy as they want (remember, no supplement can fix a terrible diet), but they will help the body digest small amounts that might occur because of cross-contamination or accidental exposure. If you'd like to have a direct link to learn more about these products, scan this QR code to get access to those two links.

3. Look over the best practices to avoid accidental exposure. Are there any changes you need to make to help prevent exposure from occurring?

CHAPTER 8:

What About Supplements?

I tried them all.

> Magnesium? Check.
> Essential oils? Check.
> Fish oil? Check.
> CBD? Check.

Other supplements that claimed they would improve focus? Check.

The amount of money and time that I spent researching and then trying supplements and other natural treatments for ADHD could have put both of my children through college. I joined Facebook groups for caregivers of children with ADHD. I followed ADHD experts on Instagram. I dug into the research online. I bought books from experts. I read everything I could get my hands on.

As you can imagine, there were constant "suggestions" from others. "Try this supplement. It worked wonders on my son …" "Try this one. My cousin's nephew is like a different kid now that he's taking it." People wanted to help. I know that now. But it was discouraging to constantly try new "miracle cures" that didn't work for us.

I wanted peace. I wanted happiness. And yet, no matter what I tried, nothing made one bit of difference.

Every time I learned about a new supplement, I was certain it was going to be "the one." THIS supplement would finally give us some relief. I'd allow myself to hope again, to think that maybe—just maybe—we could be happy.

As a child, did you ever imagine what your family would look like someday? I did. I pictured me and my spouse and our children. In all of my pictures, we were happy. There were smiles on our faces, and joy shone out of us so much that it was obvious to anyone looking that we loved one another. That picture-perfect family of my imagination didn't fit with my reality. In real life, we weren't happy. Tantrums and yelling were the norm for us, not smiles and joy.

At the end of one particularly trying day, I fell into bed beside my husband, tears threatening to spill out, and said the truth I had been thinking but had never said aloud before. "I don't even like him." Then the tears fell as shame flooded my face. What kind of mother doesn't like her own child? What kind of mother thinks deep down—in the places where no one else can see—that she obviously isn't cut out for this whole motherhood thing? I wanted a different life, one that didn't involve ADHD.

As a result, when someone told me about a new supplement that worked for them, I let myself imagine those pictures again. I let myself hope that things could improve. I allowed myself to think that maybe we could be happy as a family.

Sadly, most of the supplements didn't change anything for us. At least, not at first and in the way I was using them.

Have you been there?

If you have, then you probably know all about the disappointment that comes when the "miracle" supplement doesn't work. Or worse, when it actually creates more symptoms than there were before!

That's what happened to me with magnesium. After learning about how beneficial magnesium can be for children with ADHD, I was certain it was our missing piece, that once my son began taking it regularly, we would get some relief. Imagine my surprise when that didn't happen, when instead of relief we saw more aggression. More hyperactivity. More defiance. Our "miracle" wasn't a miracle at all. It was just another setback.

Have you been there?

When trying to find a supplement to help reduce ADHD symptoms naturally, the sheer number of options out there can be STAGGERING. I felt like I was constantly researching THIS supplement or THAT supplement and trying to figure out which one would actually work for my son. It was like a blindfold game of Pin the Tail on the Donkey at a kid's birthday party. I was aimlessly trying to hit the mark but really had no idea where I was or what I was doing.

Sadly, many families I speak with have done the same thing, aimlessly trying supplement after supplement and hoping to see results but being disappointed time and time again.

In the pages ahead, we'll learn about the best supplements for ADHD, the ones that often do help reduce ADHD symptoms in many children. Before we do that, though, it's important to understand three critical pitfalls of supplementation. Let's dive in.

Pitfall #1: Blind Supplementation

When I first started using supplements to help my son with ADHD, I did what many families do: used "blind supplementation." You won't find "blind supplementation" in a dictionary, because it's a term I made up. Blind supplementation refers to the blindfolded, Pin the Tail on the Donkey method that most of us use to choose supplements for our children. We spin in circles, desperately trying to figure out what's going to hit the target. As we spin, we listen to people all around us telling us what we should do—which way we should go. Eventually, we take a shot and hope it lands.

Blind supplementation is what I did for years, and it's what many families still do. Blind supplementation is what happens when we hear that a supplement worked for X, so we try it and hope it'll work for us too. It is supplementation without lab testing first.

There's nothing inherently wrong with blind supplementation, as long as it is being done safely, using only the prescribed amounts. For some families, blind supplementation works. They take a shot and it lands on the bullseye. They are the lucky ones. These are probably the families who are speaking up in Facebook groups and other support groups with their "suggestions" on what to try. They saw success and can't help but share it with others, assuming other people will see the same results they do. Unfortunately, blind supplementation doesn't work for many families. Many of us—myself included—end up trying way too many supplements, with way too few positive results.

I can hear the question forming in the minds of many of you reading this: "If blind supplementation doesn't work, then what does? Does that mean the only time someone should try supplementation is after lab testing?" In an ideal world, if money were no object, then I would suggest everyone do functional lab testing before trying any supplements. We'll get into functional lab testing more in a later chapter, so don't worry if you're not sure what this entails right now. You will soon!

Lab testing removes the guesswork from the process. We're not blindly spinning in circles, hoping to land on a supplement that our child's body needs. Rather, we are using the test results to see what vitamins and minerals are missing and then filling in the gaps.

If you think lab testing is the right direction for your family and would like guidance along the way, my team and I would love to help you. Scan this QR code to schedule a phone call with us. There are no obligations with this call. We will simply explain the lab testing process and discuss with you whether testing is the right course of action for your family.

Lab testing is ideal. But that's not the world we live in. Functional lab testing can be expensive and isn't often covered by insurance, so it's not always an option. In that case, trial and error is the way to go.

If that's where you find yourself today—thinking lab testing isn't for you—I don't want you to do the same blindfolded, Pin the Tail on the Donkey kind of supplementation I did. I want you to take the blindfold off. There is some trial and error with the supplements I'm going to suggest in this chapter, but I will *only* suggest supplements that are proven to be effective. I don't want you wasting your time and your money on supplements that don't work for most people.

Pitfall #2: The Miracle Pill

Supplements can be very effective and healing, but supplements can never be the be-all and end-all for ADHD symptoms. I have spoken to many caregivers who want a simple pill to "fix" their child's symptoms. They want something to make all of the challenges go away. I've been there too. This is exactly what motivated me to spend thousands of dollars on a variety of supplements that promised relief.

The hard reality, though, is that if a child is still consuming large amounts of inflammatory, processed foods, he or she won't likely see a noticeable improvement using ANY supplement. That's because the body is still being pounded by inflammation, and inflammation, as we learned in an earlier chapter, affects much more than just the gut. It affects the entire body. Children cannot function at their best if the diet is not cleaned up.

For that reason, food should always come first. For about half of the families I work with, once the diet is changed, supplementation is not necessary at all. Diet alone can provide them with the relief they need. For other families, supplementation is necessary to provide full reduction of ADHD symptoms. Even for these families, though, if they ONLY supplement and don't change the diet, it won't work. Food MUST come first. It is a vital—100 percent essential—part of natural ADHD symptom reduction. You can't supplement your way out of a poor diet.

> **YOU CAN'T SUPPLEMENT YOUR WAY OUT OF A POOR DIET.**

My fear with supplementation is that families might view supplements as miracle cures, thinking they can continue to eat terrible food as long as they are taking the supplement. It won't work that way. In order for supplementation to be effective, it cannot be done alone. Food must come first.

Food is our primary tool for symptom reduction. Supplementation is the support that helps us along the way. If someone tries to reverse these two, making supplementation the primary tool and food the support, they will not succeed.

Food is the lead role; supplements are the supporting actors. In a play, if you try to force a supporting actor into the lead role, be prepared for a disaster. He won't know the lines. He'll miss cues. That critic in the audience will not be impressed. So it is with food and supplementation. They need to stay in their assigned roles. Food is the lead. Supplements are the support.

Pitfall #3: One Size Fits All

A third pitfall with supplementation is that many people assume if a supplement works for one child with ADHD, it will work for their own child as well. I definitely fell into this trap with my son. I mistakenly assumed that because magnesium worked for other families that it was guaranteed to work for ours. When it didn't, I was crushed.

Every child is a bio-individual. Unique. Unlike anyone else on this planet. One supplement that works well for one child might not have much of an effect on another child, or it might even have a negative effect. That's because each child is his or her own individual and needs different things, based on diet and genetic makeup.

I often compare it to baking. Certain recipes call for certain ingredients. The ingredients for each recipe are essential to a delicious finished product, and you can't always swap out one ingredient for a different ingredient and assume it will work the same. If you've already started swapping out your regular flour for gluten-free varieties, you probably know exactly what I mean. It can be very tricky to find the right combination when working with substitutions. Sometimes, you might get lucky with a substitution and end up with an equally delicious finished product. Other times, though, the substitutions can lead to baking disasters.

Have you ever accidentally left out baking powder from a bread or other baked good? A few months ago, I was making breakfast muffins for my family and accidentally left out the baking powder. The muffins were somewhat edible (though I'm using the word "somewhat" very loosely), but the texture was terrible. It was like eating a piece of banana-flavored rubber. The reason the muffins were so bad was because they were missing a key ingredient.

Our bodies have certain vitamins and minerals they need to function at their best, but without lab testing, we have no way of knowing which vitamins might be missing. Therefore, when we supplement we might get lucky and give the body an ingredient it needs, or we might overload it with something it already has plenty of.

For supplementation to be most effective, it needs to be tailored to each individual child. Remember, this book is not intended as a substitute for the medical advice of physicians, so it's always best to chat with your child's doctor.[46] We'll discuss functional lab testing more in a later chapter. For now, keep in mind as you read about supplements that some of them might not give you the results you are hoping for. Don't give up! That means your child has a different ingredient that he or she needs. Stick with me, and we'll get you there!

Top Supplements for Children with ADHD

If blind supplementation isn't always effective AND if there is no miracle cure AND if what works for one child might not work for mine, why bother? Why even attempt to find a supplement to help?

In reality, supplementation can be a critical supporting factor in reducing ADHD symptoms. As I said, I do suggest lab testing first, if possible (and we will discuss that more in a later chapter), but even if lab testing isn't an option for your family, there are still some supplements that can be beneficial. Remember, though, there are exceptions. Every child is unique. If one of these supplements does not help your child, don't quit trying to find something that will.

Supplement #1: Fish Oil

The first supplement I recommend for children with ADHD is a good quality fish oil for omega-3 and omega-6 fatty acids. Omega-3 and omega-6 fatty acids are polyunsaturated fatty acids that our bodies cannot make on their own. That means the only way we obtain these types of fat is through diet (or, with regard to our current discussion, through supplementation).

Fats have gotten an unnecessarily bad name in our culture in recent years because of the misconception that all fats are bad. In reality, fat is NOT the enemy. Rather, fat is something our bodies and brains need to function and survive.

Getting enough healthy fat is critical for growth and development, especially for our compromised kids. Here are a few reasons we need healthy fats:

- Fat builds the brain
- Fat helps with cell signaling and repair
- Fat produces hormones our bodies need
- Fat absorbs vitamins that are critical to our health and development
- Fat produces healthy skin
- Fat helps maintain our body temperature
- Fat serves as a source of fuel for our bodies
- Fat protects vital organs by holding them in place and cushioning them

As you can see from this list, fat isn't the problem! Fat can be very beneficial for our bodies and especially for our brains! One of the best fats for brain health is polyunsaturated fat (like omega-3 and omega-6 fatty acids).

Omega-3 fatty acids can be found in oily fish such as salmon, trout, mackerel, tuna, and sardines, in nuts such as almonds, walnuts, hazelnuts, and pecans, and in seeds such as chia, flax, and pumpkin. Omega-6 fatty acids are found in many plant-based oils.

Omega-3 and omega-6 fatty acids are meant to be in a one-to-one ratio in the body. Unfortunately, because of the Western diet, the amount of omega-6 fatty acids in our bodies has reached unprecedented proportions and results in inflammation, blood pressure issues, and heart disorders. In contrast, omega-3 fatty acids, which come from a Mediterranean diet, are typically extremely low in Americans.[47]

This deficiency of omega-3 fatty acids is correlated to ADHD in children. Paul Montgomery, D.Phil., a researcher at the University of Oxford in England, gave school-age children fish oil supplementation for three months to help boost their omega-3 fatty acid intake. At the end of that time, he found that those taking the supplements showed improvement in behavior, as well as in reading and spelling. He concluded in *Pediatrics* that "a lack of certain polyunsaturated fatty acids may contribute to dyslexia and attention-deficit/hyperactivity disorder."[48] Research[49] suggests this deficiency in omega-3 fatty acids can be improved by incorporating foods that naturally contain fatty acids such as fish and nuts. Unfortunately, many children refuse to eat these types of foods, preferring to stick with other, more kid-friendly dishes. Because of this, supplementation is often the way to go for children.

Supplement #2: Probiotics

Do you remember in a previous chapter where we discussed the gut-brain connection? As noted, the brain has many areas that are involved in gut function, but one of the main areas is the frontal lobe. The frontal lobe talks to the gut via nerve branches and two-way chemical messengers. It is involved in things like attention, focus, executive function, planning, organizing, and problem-solving; issues with these capacities are common to many of our children with ADHD.

When we ensure that our children's guts are functioning well, we simultaneously ensure their frontal lobes are functioning well too. That's why probiotics can be so beneficial for children with ADHD. Probiotics can be found naturally in kombucha, dark chocolate, and fermented foods, and they can also come in supplement form.

Research[50] shows that probiotics that contain a certain type of gut bacteria can reduce inflammation in the body,[51] help detoxify, reduce anxiety, improve mood, and also protect the body against the damaging mental and physical effects of stress.[52]

Supplement #3: Magnesium

Magnesium and I have a love-hate relationship. When I first heard about how effective magnesium can be at reducing ADHD symptoms, I was sure it was *the one!* Magnesium was going to be the "miracle cure" in our family. You already know how that turned out. It wasn't. There is no such thing as a miracle cure. There is no one-size-fits-all supplement that is going to "fix" ADHD. For my son, magnesium actually exacerbated his symptoms. He was worse off taking this supplement than he was taking nothing!

So why am I even telling you about magnesium if it worked so poorly for my son? Why even include it in this list of my top supplements for ADHD? Because science speaks loudly about how effective it can be for some children and because I have seen how effective it can be for many of the families I work with. Remember, every child is unique. Just because magnesium wasn't our game-changer doesn't mean it won't be yours.

Magnesium is used in more than 300 biochemical processes in the body, and it is an important element that supports muscles, helps with relaxation, aids restful sleep, keeps hormonal balance, keeps the heartbeat steady, regulates blood glucose levels, and aids in the production of energy. Stress depletes magnesium levels, so if a child is already low in magnesium and experiences stress, that anxiety can make their magnesium levels even lower. It's a vicious cycle, but one that can be supported through eating magnesium-rich foods like spinach, asparagus, cabbage, avocado, bananas, seeds, nuts, peas, broccoli, dark chocolate, or oily fish. It can also be supported through supplementation.

Many caregivers find that magnesium makes a surprising difference in their kids' anxiety or depression, aids in sleep, and also reduces hyperactivity. Research suggests that children with ADHD often have low magnesium levels, and using supplements can have a calming effect on behavior[53] and reduce insomnia, agitation, and muscle cramps. With magnesium, it's important to remember that it can take a couple of weeks to up to a month to build up in the body, so don't expect immediate results.

Supplement #4: Vitamin D

A fourth supplement that is often effective in reducing ADHD symptoms is vitamin D. It is especially effective when taken with a supplement of omega-3 fatty acids. That's because these nutrients play a vital role in our serotonin production. Serotonin is our feel-good hormone and is closely tied to issues with behavior, appetite, sleep, digestion, and memory—all things that many children with ADHD battle.

Vitamin D also helps reduce inflammation in the body. As we discussed in an earlier chapter, inflammation in the body affects much more than just gut health. Once that inflammation reaches the brain, it can also create behavior issues, hyperactivity, anger issues, problems with memory, and so on.

One of the best natural ways to get more vitamin D is to get outside in the sunlight, but since this is not always possible, a vitamin D supplement can be very beneficial. Other food sources for vitamin D include oily fish, cod liver oil, mushrooms, and egg yolks.

Supplement #5: Vitamin C

Vitamin C is well known for its benefits when battling sickness, but many people don't realize that it's also a crucial vitamin for children's health and development. Vitamin C acts as an antioxidant and helps reduce free radical damage and inflammation in the body, which is the key to reducing symptoms in our children. It also influences the neurotransmitter dopamine in the brain. Dopamine, as you might remember, is associated with mood, social development, and sleep.

The body actually doesn't make vitamin C on its own, so it's important that diet be rich in foods containing this particular vitamin. Some foods that are high in vitamin C include guava, yellow and green bell peppers, kiwi, strawberries, raspberries, blueberries, cranberries, oranges, lemons, papaya, broccoli, kale, tomato, cauliflower, and mango. Supplementation can also help bridge the gap when the diet is lacking.

Supplement #6: Zinc

Zinc is a powerful antioxidant. It boosts cell growth and development and improves immunity. It also aids in the creation of neurotransmitters such as serotonin and dopamine—those happy, feel-good neurotransmitters we talked about earlier—which are associated with improved mood, social development, and sleep.

Another reason zinc is so important is because of how it relates to copper in the body. When zinc is low, copper gets high, and this can lead to a deficiency of dopamine. Because of this, balancing out that copper/zinc ratio is really important, and the usual way to do this is to increase zinc.

Zinc is also important when it comes to things like brain development, auditory processing, language processing, sensory processing, eye contact, muscle tone, and so on. Research[54] has found that zinc supplementation can be helpful in reducing ADHD symptoms.

Supplement #7: Iron

Many people only associate low levels of iron with anemia, but iron is critical for optimal brain function. Some researchers also believe that low levels of iron can be an underlying stressor for ADHD. In one particular study, iron-deficient ADHD children were given iron supplements. These children saw improvement in their ADHD symptoms, as compared to the children who did not receive the supplementation.[55]

Some foods that are naturally high in iron include lean beef and poultry, oysters and shellfish, cashews, pumpkin seeds, quinoa, spinach, broccoli, and dark chocolate. If you believe your child might have low levels of iron, consider whether supplementation might be beneficial.

What About Herbs?

I have also found several herbs to be very beneficial for many children with ADHD. The first herb I recommend often is *Rhodiola rosea*. Don't let the long name scare you! Rhodiola is simply an herb that grows in both Europe and Asia. Its roots are believed to help people adjust to stress. As children with ADHD often struggle to cope with emotional distress, this herb can be beneficial for them. People have been using rhodiola to help with depression, anxiety, and fatigue for centuries. Today, this herb is a widely used supplement. You can read more about it through the link at the end of the book.[56]

OPCs (short for oligomeric proanthocyanidins) are plant-based compounds I often recommend. OPCs are derived from plants such as peaches, blueberries, cranberries, grapes, and others. Plants create these OPCs to fight against environmental toxins, but they can be very beneficial for humans. There are some studies that suggest these compounds, when ingested through supplementation, can be beneficial for brain function, in particular with regard to executive function, concentration, and focus.[57]

Finally, ginkgo and ginseng can also be helpful for children with ADHD. *ADDitude* magazine explained the unique benefits of these two herbs this way: "They act like stimulants without the side effects. Typically, adults and children who take ginkgo and ginseng improve on ADHD rating scales, and are less impulsive and distractible."[58]

With all of these supplements and herbs, it's important to remember that none of them can "fix" a child's ADHD. It's also important to remember that no one supplement can serve as the be-all and end-all for symptom reduction. No matter what supplements or herbs are being taken, diet is still the most important piece of natural symptom reduction.

The supplements and herbs covered in this chapter, though, can still serve as great "supporting actors" to diet. They are some of the top supplements for children with ADHD because of how effective they often are at reducing common ADHD symptoms. As mentioned, there is always a chance that some children might not necessarily need one or more of these supplements, based on their individual bodies and what they are already getting from diet, so always consult your health practitioner before starting any new supplement.

There's no way to know exactly which supplements your child needs without functional lab testing. If you'd like to know more about how lab testing works, scan this QR code to schedule a free call with my team. There are no obligations with this call. We will simply explain the lab testing process and discuss with you whether or not testing is the right course of action for your family.

Chapter Highlights

- Supplementation can be effective at reducing ADHD symptoms in children. There are, however, three significant pitfalls to keep in mind:
    - "Blind supplementation" is not always effective. A much more effective strategy is to remove the blindfold and target supplementation based on a child's specific deficiencies.
    - You can't supplement your way out of a poor diet. Food is the foundation of every effective treatment plan. Supplementation plays the supporting role, not the lead.
    - Just because a supplement works for one child does not guarantee it will work for another. Every child is unique, so it's important to understand there is no one-size-fits-all supplement.
- The following supplements can be effective at reducing ADHD symptoms in children:
    - Fish oil
    - Probiotic
    - Magnesium
    - Vitamin D
    - Vitamin C
    - Zinc
    - Iron
- Herbs can also be effective at reducing ADHD symptoms, especially the following herbs:
    - *Rhodiola rosea*
    - OPC
    - Ginkgo and ginseng

Action Steps

1. Think through the three pitfalls of supplementation:

    ▷ Supplementing blindly

    ▷ Hoping to find the miracle cure

    ▷ Assuming one size fits all

    Which of these three have you fallen into before? What steps can you take moving forward to make sure you don't fall into them again?

2. Consider whether you would like to try any of the supplements listed in this chapter. If you decide to try one (or several), remember to start low and go slow. Start with one supplement at a time, at the lowest possible dose. Slowly increase until you reach the full dose for your child's weight. Then, once your child has been on that supplement for three days with no adverse reactions, it is safe to introduce a second supplement. Never begin two supplements at the same time, in case there are adverse reactions like an increase in challenging behaviors, rashes, stomach pain, changes in stool, or tiredness. Start with one, slowly increase, wait a few days, and then introduce another.

    Also remember, this book is not intended as a substitute for the medical advice of physicians. The reader should consult a physician in matters relating to health and particularly with respect to symptoms that may require diagnosis or medical attention.

CHAPTER 9:

But What About ...? Common Obstacles and How to Overcome Them, Part 1

"He only eats a total of five foods." Rachel's words surprised me. I had worked with picky eaters in the past, but never this picky. She went on to share their family's story.

Rachel's son, Landon, caught a respiratory syncytial virus (RSV) at age two. That RSV quickly developed into asthma. Landon had to take daily medications for his asthma and allergies and was still sick nearly every month. It was during that time his picky eating developed. They tried food therapy. No progress. They tried play therapy. Nothing. They considered medication, but Rachel didn't want to go down that road yet. She wanted to try something more natural—something that wouldn't be an up-and-down battle as her son grew and developed.

That's what led her to find me and my program. Landon didn't only have picky eating challenges, though. He also had anger and rage issues. His meltdowns were a daily occurrence. He was becoming more and more out of control as each day passed. Rachel was desperate. Miserable. When we spoke on the phone, she told me that Landon couldn't even make eye contact most of the time. He couldn't carry on a conversation. He was so different from the child she knew he could be, and she needed help.

To be honest, though, I second-guessed my ability to help this family. I had worked with other picky eaters, but none this picky. I lay in bed that night and voiced my concerns to my husband, Ben. "What if I can't get him eating a more diverse diet? What if this is the first child that I really can't help?" Ben wrapped his arms around me and told me exactly what I needed to hear: that I could do this and that we could help their family.

In the pages ahead, I'm going to be honest with you about the challenges you might face with this lifestyle change. I wish I could tell you it's easy. I wish I could say you won't face challenges like picky eating or family members who don't support your decision. I can't. The reality is, this way of living goes against the grain.

People won't always agree with your choices. Some of them will probably be very vocal with their disagreements. Doing something that is different isn't always easy, but it is worth it. Visionary, public speaker, and author Mark Shayler said, "Change the status quo or become it." I don't want to become the status quo, and since you're reading this book, I bet you don't either. I don't want to battle high cholesterol, heart disease, and cancer. I don't want my kids to become the status quo either. If we want to be different, we have to live different lives. We can't be comfortable doing what everyone else is doing. And because of this, we will face opposition.

In the pages ahead, I'm going to help you prepare yourself for how to deal with some of the most common challenges families face when changing the diets of their children. These challenges include picky eating as well as unsupportive (or downright oppositional) family, friends, or school staff. In the next chapter, we'll look at a couple of other obstacles many families face. Let's dive in.

Obstacle #1: Picky Eating

What do most children eat in this country? Chicken nuggets? Pizza? Hot dogs? Grilled cheese sandwiches? French fries and potato chips? The food industry has trained us to believe that children will only eat "kid foods." Children won't eat kale, brussels sprouts, broccoli, or anything green that grows in the ground. They might eat fruit, but vegetables? Not a chance.

I'm here to tell you that's not the truth. The food industry might try to tell us our children won't eat "adult" food, but they will. I've seen it time and time again as children move past their picky eating and begin to like—not just endure or tolerate, but actually like—vegetables. One parent shared this win in our private Facebook group:

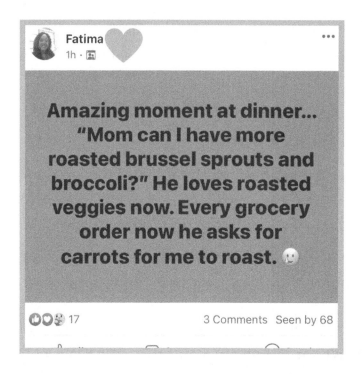

No matter how picky your child might be, there is hope! There are strategies you can use to get them to eat "non-kid" foods. Let's take a look at a few of them.

Picky Eating Strategy #1: Make Mealtimes Fun

The first picky eating tip I share with every caregiver in my program is to make mealtimes fun. Try to be calm and upbeat during mealtime. The last thing caregivers of children with ADHD need is yet another power struggle. Unfortunately, that's often what happens with new foods IF we aren't intentional about making meals fun and engaging for our children.

Mealtimes used to be the WORST time of the day in my family. In fact, they got so bad that sometimes I just wanted to hide in the cupboard instead of sitting down with my family. After I removed our gluten/dairy/soy staples, the battles became even worse. My children wouldn't try anything new, and

I refused to serve the old foods they were used to. It was a nightly war zone that often ended with me in tears. It was only after I made an intentional effort to make meals fun again that my children began trying some of the new foods I set on the table.

I used to encourage them to crunch their food like a bunny rabbit, or lick the new food like a puppy dog. We would all laugh, and it took the tension out of dinner time. For older kids, take a joke book to the table, sharing a joke before the meal and for every new food they try.

Another way to make mealtime fun AND to work toward breaking those picky eating habits is to do a family challenge. To do this, begin by having a family meeting to talk about the importance of eating a variety of foods for our bodies to make them healthy. At this meeting, introduce the family food challenge. Work together to choose a reward that the entire family will enjoy. Then, take turns choosing one new food each week. Trying more than one new food at a time can make the experience overwhelming or stressful. Write your chosen food down on a note in your kitchen.

Then, every night that week, offer the new food before dinner. Ask everyone in the family to examine it, lick it, smell it, and taste it and then share their observations. Do this for seven nights in a row. Why seven? Because it can take 7 to 15 and sometimes up to 20 times for a palate to adjust to a new food. Just because children say they don't like something the first time they try it does not mean they won't like it the 15th time they try it!

Each night that your family (and that includes everyone in the family—not just the child you are working with) tries the new food, put a checkmark or a tally mark beside the food on the note. When you reach a certain number of marks (this could be 2 or 5 or 7 or 20—whatever you think your children need to motivate them), reward the entire family. This could be a dinner out or ice cream (dairy-free, of course) or a family game night or a night at the movies. These family challenges do two things: 1) they make dinner fun again, and 2) they get the entire family involved in the picky eating battle.

Picky Eating Strategy #2: Be Aware of WHEN You Are Introducing New Foods

A second strategy to remember when introducing new food is to be aware of WHEN you are offering the new food. Don't give your child new foods when they aren't very hungry. By introducing new foods at a time when your child is hungry, you are ensuring they will be more open and willing to taste them. Is your child starving when he comes home from school? Offer the new food then, as a snack. Does your child take medication that makes her not hungry for lunch? Then avoid introducing a new food during lunch.

Keep in mind, however, that it's a good idea to pair new foods with at least one familiar food that your child enjoys. Doing this will ensure weight does not drop too much. It will also ensure your child doesn't get HANGRY if he refuses to try the new food you are introducing.

Picky Eating Strategy #3: Use Food Chaining

Food chaining is a technique by which a parent changes the way that a food item is served. It involves changing the shape, seasoning, or cooking method of a food that a child already likes, slowly transitioning them to a healthier variety.

For example, think about a potato. Most children probably like french fries, but there are MUCH healthier ways to cook a potato. If a parent were to remove french fries from the diet abruptly and replace them with baked potatoes, most children would not like the change. Some would downright refuse to even try the baked potato! Food chaining can help make this transition easier.

Begin by offering a healthier french fry. Rather than fries at a restaurant that are deep-fried in vegetable oil and coated with a ton of preservatives, buy a bag of frozen french fries at the grocery store that don't have all the added junk in them, and cook those at home. Once your child is used to these, try making homemade french fries in your oven or air fryer using a sliced potato, olive or avocado oil, salt, and pepper. Try this for several days. Then, once your child has adjusted to these, make another slight variation by using sweet potatoes instead or by changing the seasoning. Keep introducing the same food every few days, but change up the shape, seasoning, and preparation. You can deep fry, pan fry, make into mash or tots, add spices, or combine with sweet potato mash. Each of these small steps adjusts your child's palate and opens it up to different textures and flavors.

Another common food we often use food chaining with is chicken nuggets. Most children enjoy chicken nuggets. Caregivers can use food chaining with chicken nuggets to get them eating grilled chicken breasts. Follow these steps:

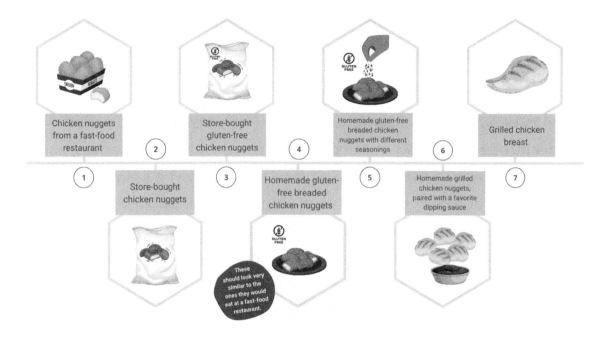

Don't change the food your child enjoys; change the way you serve it! Change the texture and the seasonings. Include herbs and spices. It's all about changing things slowly and carefully, starting with a food that your child already loves.

Picky Eating Strategy #4: Slowly Adapt Taste Buds

"She won't eat any of the dairy-free yogurts I have bought. She hates them all!" Hannah had tried all of the varieties: yogurt made with coconut milk, almond milk, cashew milk, and oat milk. Her daughter hated them all (though, to be fair, some of them she refused to even try). "What am I supposed to do now?" she asked us on a coaching call one Thursday afternoon.

We advised Hannah to do one of two things: 1) stop eating yogurt altogether for a few months, allowing the body to "forget" the taste of regular yogurt and then reintroduce it with a dairy-free variety after a few months, or 2) slowly adapt the taste buds.

To slowly adapt the taste buds, begin by mixing three-fourths of the dairy yogurt with one-fourth of the non-dairy yogurt. Do this for a few days. Then, once she has adjusted to this, change the ratios to one-half dairy yogurt mixed with one-half non-dairy yogurt. Then, a few days later, change the ratios again to one-fourth dairy yogurt mixed with three-fourths non-dairy. This strategy works really well with yogurt, but also with milk. If the product you are needing to introduce is a liquid, consider using this method to slowly adapt the taste buds.

Picky Eating Strategy #5: Consider Whether Zinc Could Be a Contributing Factor

Many people don't realize that zinc deficiency can be a contributing factor to picky eating. Zinc plays an important role in brain development, auditory processing, language processing, sensory processing, regulating the immune functions, eye contact, muscle tone, and so on. There is research that suggests that zinc plays a crucial role in regulating how neurons in our brain communicate with one another,[59, 60] affecting how our memories are formed and how we learn. It makes sense, then, that a deficiency in zinc can be very closely correlated with disorders that affect the brain.

Zinc deficiency can actually cause a loss of taste buds and affect the way that our brain processes the taste of something. Once this has happened, many foods can actually taste terrible or even offensive. As the levels of zinc diminish, the way food tastes gets worse, and then aversions to food obviously increase. This can happen with any food but seems most common with vegetables or foods with unique textures, smells, or colors. What results is the child then starts to limit the food, and it becomes a vicious cycle. What might have started as zinc deficiency quickly becomes a habit, and habits are very hard to break and a lot of times they can get worse.

The good news is that zinc levels can easily be changed through diet or supplementation. Foods that are high in zinc include beef, spinach, pumpkin seeds, and shrimp, but if a child is severely deficient in zinc, supplementation might be necessary. Zinc levels can be measured in the blood or in the hair. Testing before supplementing is always the best course of action because that ensures we are only giving a child what his or her body actually needs.

That's why I love that there is a quick home test caregivers can do themselves. It is called the zinc assay taste test. It is quick and easy. Caregivers provide their children with a teaspoon full of zinc assay, and the children will experience varying tastes based on the body's current level of zinc. If it tastes immediately unpleasant, the child most likely has optimal zinc levels. If the child says it is tasteless or tastes like water, they are likely very deficient in zinc.

If you would like to know more information about this at-home zinc assay test, scan this QR code to gain access to the link to the zinc assay test we use, as well as a chart that explains exactly how to interpret your child's response to the zinc.

Picky Eating Strategy #6: Change the Diet, Change the Taste Buds

Picky eating is—without a doubt—the most common challenge families face when adapting their child's diet. Recently, I was thinking back to when we started on this journey with my son, fighting his ADHD symptoms with food.

We used to struggle so much, not just with his behavior and tantrums but also with his eating.

We used to battle at literally EVERY SINGLE MEAL. It was stressful and unpleasant. I felt like a failure as a mom. I wanted to disappear most nights. But then, as I began changing the foods we ate, I started seeing his palate open up as well—slowly at first, but then more rapidly.

What I learned is that picky eating and inflammation go hand in hand. When you start reducing inflammation in the body, brain, and gut by changing the foods your child eats, their palate opens up as a result. I like to think of it like this:

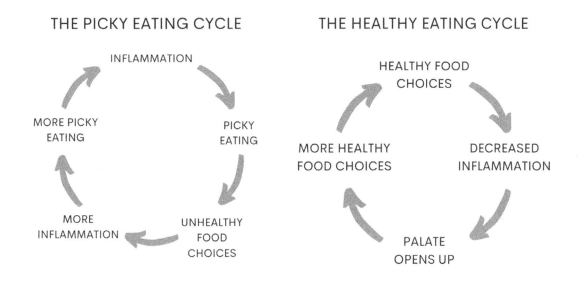

There are two options as far as picky eating is concerned. You can either continue on the picky-eating cycle, leading to more inflammation, more bad eating habits, and even more picky eating, OR you can start using the strategies covered in this chapter to slowly adjust your child's diet to healthier options, reducing inflammation in the process and opening up their palate as a result.

Where Rachel and Landon Are Now

Rachel was the first parent I had ever spoken to who honestly made me question my ability to help. Her son Landon only ate a total of five foods! FIVE! When we agreed to work together, I put on a brave face and hoped she couldn't see through it. If she knew I wasn't sure I could help them, she wouldn't believe it was possible either, so I put on my big girl pants and hid my self-doubt. We got to work, and I'm happy to share that he now eats more than 100 different foods!

Even though both Rachel and I worried about Landon's picky eating, she took the plunge and is so glad she did. "I have my child back," she told me a few weeks ago. Landon used to have issues with anger and out-of-control rage. Daily meltdowns. He couldn't control himself at all. Plus, he was sick monthly!

Now, he's healthy and thriving. His daily tantrums are almost completely gone. He can sit still and look her in the eye (which he could never do before). He's eating more than 100 foods! He went from 5 to more than 100 in just a few short months, using the same strategies in this chapter! If Rachel can do it, I know you can do it too! No more excuses. You've got this!

If you feel like you'd like some additional support with this, I would be happy to chat with you about potentially working with my team. Scan this QR code to set up a free phone call to chat about our process: how it works, what we ask of you, what you get from us, and so on. No obligations. Just a phone call to see if we are the right fit and to discuss how we can help you overcome picky eating problems.

Obstacle #2: Unsupportive Family/Friends

Next to picky eating, unsupportive family members or friends is the second-most common obstacle families face when overhauling their child's diet. What do you do when you want to change your child's diet but your partner, other family members, or friends aren't on board? How do you handle the criticism? How do you convince them to go along with the changes when they don't think they're necessary, don't want to spend the money on healthier food options, or don't want to take the time to make such a big change?

In the next few pages, I'm going to share some strategies to help with this. Let's get going!

Support-Winning Strategy #1: Show Them the Science

Regardless of the specific hang-up your family member or friend is facing, I have found in working with close to one thousand families that one of the best ways to convince the unconvinced is to share the research. The truth (which you already read in the beginning of this book) is that science is far from silent on the topic of the gut-brain connection!

Many people don't support dietary changes because they don't realize how effective they can be at managing ADHD symptoms. It's not so much a lack of support as it is a lack of knowledge. Use this book as a resource to discuss the facts about natural ADHD symptom reduction with them.

When my son's doctor suggested that fourth medication and I decided enough was enough, I began looking for other solutions. To be honest, I was skeptical too. I assumed natural strategies wouldn't work. After all, I had already tried SO MANY THINGS and didn't want to waste any more money on something that wasn't going to work. It was the science that convinced me to give it a try. When I read the Autism Research Institute study I mentioned in Chapter 1 about the effectiveness of dietary changes compared to the effectiveness of medications, I was sold!

To help you begin the conversation with your family members or friends about the science behind this approach, my team and I put together a letter for you to share with them. If you'd like a copy of this letter, scan this QR code.

Support-Winning Strategy #2: Share Your WHY with Them

For some, science is enough to change their minds about the natural approach. But it's possible that even after you share the research from this book with them—even after you explain the gut-brain connection and even after you talk about the effects of inflammation on the body—they still won't support your decision.

In that case, it might be time to share your WHY. Why are you making these changes? What challenges were you facing that led you to make this decision? They might be able to ignore the research, but they're less likely to ignore your story.

My WHY when I originally started down this road was my unhappiness and the unhappiness of my entire family. ADHD was ruining our lives. My husband and I walked on eggshells in our own home, waiting for the next meltdown from our son. We fought constantly because the tension in the house was high all the time. The medicine wasn't helping Oliver. In fact, it was creating new problems—anxiety, sleeplessness, fear, and worry.

One night, I realized I was living for bedtime. I didn't enjoy my life when I was awake. It was just too much. Realizing that was an eye-opener. What kind of life is it if you're just living for bedtime? If you don't enjoy spending time with your family? If the only thing you look forward to is sleep? That's not the life I wanted to have, so I made the changes necessary to get a different life. THAT is my WHY. What is yours?

Why are you wanting to make these changes? Why are you reading this book? When we are little, many of us grow up imagining our futures. We have this image in our head of what our family life might look like. What is that picture for you? My guess is that your current day-to-day reality isn't matching up to that picture. Otherwise, you probably wouldn't be reading this book.

I get it. My picture wasn't matching up for a long time either. At my lowest, there was even a time when I thought my picture-perfect family was impossible. *Maybe if I were different*, or *maybe if my child were different*, I remember thinking.

But then we changed the foods we ate, and that picture started becoming closer and closer to reality. Of course, we still have our struggles, like any family, but we are happy. We have become that family I always imagined we could be. I want that for you too!

I understand how hard it is when your family or friends aren't on board, but trust me when I tell you that the hard conversations are worth it! I would hate for you to be in the exact same position one year from now or, even worse, several years from now, when you can make changes today and see real results, sometimes in a few short weeks.

When people learn your WHY—when they hear your story and when they see your tears—they're more willing to support you and help you succeed. Even if they don't think it will work, many of them will help, simply because they love you and they understand it's important to you.

Support-Winning Strategy #3: Make It Easy

In my experience, when families use Support-Winning Strategy #1 and Support-Winning Strategy #2, most family members and friends will support their decision. There could, however, be someone out there reading this book whose family remains resistant—even after trying these two strategies. What can you do then?

In that case, it's best to make it easy for them. Do the work so they don't have to. Any time your child is with this particular family member or friend, provide the food you want your child to eat. If they want to take your child out to eat, give them a list of foods your child can eat at that restaurant. Send groceries to their house that are gluten-, dairy-, and soy-free. Pack snacks, drinks, and dinners.

Yes, it's a lot of work for you. Yes, sometimes it might make you wonder if it's even worth it. Let me reassure you, it's totally worth it! It's much better to put in the work on the front end than to deal with regression in behavior after eating unapproved foods. You will not get to where you want to go if you have a little gluten or dairy here or there because you're never really giving the body a chance to fully mend itself.

Some children take MONTHS to reduce those inflammatory responses in their bodies. The work you put in on the front end to make sure your child doesn't get a "cheat day" with a friend or family member is what will enable you to see real results.

Support-Winning Strategy #4: Let the Transformation Speak for Itself

In my experience, there is ONE thing that nearly always convinces a family member or friend to jump on board: real, lasting change! When they start to see changes in your child that they didn't even think were possible, they will quickly change their minds about this approach.

In order for that to happen, though, you have to take the first step today. Businessman and author Max De Pree said, "We cannot become what we need to be by remaining what we are." We won't see change in our child if we're not willing to make changes in their lifestyle first (and in our own, for that matter).

Obstacle #3: School Challenges

You have a plan for picky eating. You have a plan for how to approach any family members or friends who don't agree with natural solutions for ADHD. Now, what about your child's school?

As I write, more than two years have passed since the COVID-19 pandemic hit the world hard. Many of us thought the pandemic would be contained to 2020, but it continued on through 2021 and into 2022. One of the by-products of the pandemic is that the United States Department of Agriculture has reimbursed schools for free meals to all students, regardless of income.

What that means is that many of us—my children included—have had the option of eating free breakfast and lunch at school. As you can imagine, this is a blessing to many families across the U.S. Not having to worry about breakfast or lunch every single day? Sign me up, right?!

Unfortunately, though schools will work with food allergies, they aren't always willing to work with families who don't have test results or doctor's notes requiring certain food eliminations. That means the school won't provide a free meal that is gluten-, dairy-, and soy-free for your child without a note from a doctor stating it is medically necessary. Instead, if you want to make sure your child isn't eating gluten, dairy, or soy at school, you will have to provide breakfast and lunch for them.

My children don't get free meals at their school, nor do the children of the families I work with. They also don't get to participate in school-provided snacks. Instead, our families provide lunches every day and comparable (though healthier) alternatives anytime the school offers a snack. It costs more, for sure. I won't deny that. For us, it's worth the money. I'd rather have a happy family than a little extra cash in my pocket or checking account. I'd rather have their health than free food. If you agree, here are some strategies I would recommend you take as you work with your child's school:

School Strategy #1: Communicate with the School

Talk to the school staff, including your child's teacher, the nurse, the cafeteria staff, and any other teachers who might need to know about your child's special dietary needs. Explain to them why you are making the changes you are making, and ask them to refrain from providing your child with any food or candy at school. Let them know you are happy to provide plenty of snacks and candy as needed throughout the school year for your child to have when other students are given snacks or treats.

School Strategy #2: Provide Food

Provide plenty of snacks for your child to keep in his or her classroom. Include a variety of options, so your child will hopefully have items similar to what is brought in by other students. Don't forget about special drinks, candy, and cupcakes or cookies for classroom birthday parties. If your child's teacher has access to a freezer, ask the teacher to store a couple of cupcakes in the freezer. These can be pulled out for your child to enjoy when other students bring birthday treats that are filled with gluten. Ask your child's teacher to choose from these when snacks are provided in the classroom.

School Strategy #3: Talk to Your Child

Talk to your child about the importance of eating foods that are gluten-, dairy-, and soy-free. Though there is a chance they will sneak food at school that they shouldn't have (we will look at this more in the next chapter), by talking with them about why you are making these changes, they will hopefully begin to buy into the process as well.

In this chapter, we have covered three common obstacles: picky eating, unsupportive family or friends, and challenges with school. In the next chapter, we'll look at two more: what to do when a child sneaks food and how to combat the expense of eating healthier. See you there!

Chapter Highlights

- These lifestyle changes aren't without challenges. Here are some of the most common challenges you might face:
    - Picky eating
    - Unsupportive family or friends
    - School challenges
- Use the following picky eating strategies:
    - Make mealtimes fun
    - Be aware of WHEN you are introducing new foods
    - Use food chaining
    - Slowly adapt taste buds
    - Consider whether zinc could be a contributing factor
    - Change the diet. Change the taste buds
- Use the following strategies to deal with unsupportive family or friends:
    - Show them the science
    - Share your WHY
    - Make it easy for them
    - Let the transformation speak for itself
- Use the following strategies to deal with challenges at school:
    - Talk to the school staff about the changes you are making
    - Personally provide any food/drinks/treats/snacks your child might need
    - Talk to your child about the importance of the changes you are making

Action Steps

1. Thinking through the picky-eating strategies in this chapter, choose one that you want to try this week. Is it a mealtime game, a family food challenge, changing the time that you introduce new foods, food chaining, or the zinc assay test? You don't have to do everything at once! Choose ONE strategy to try this week, and put it into practice.

2. Scan this QR code to gain access to the information about the zinc assay test, to schedule a free call with my team, or to grab your copy of a letter we have written for unsupportive family members to help them understand the importance of the changes we are suggesting.

3. What is your WHY? Take about ten minutes and write it down. Why are you wanting to make these changes in your family? What is your motivation?

4. Are there any family members, friends, or school staff whom you need to inform about the changes you are making? If so, put reminders on your calendar to take these necessary steps.

5. Are you packing your child's lunch for school, ensuring it is gluten-, dairy-, and soy-free? If not, start doing that this week!

6. Have you provided snacks for your child to keep at school? If not, go shopping this week for gluten-, dairy-, and soy-free snacks that you can send with your child to school. Make sure and check in periodically with your child's teacher to see if more snacks are needed for your child's stash.

CHAPTER 10:

But What About ...? Common Obstacles and How to Overcome Them, Part 2

Remember my little tirade when I tossed every product in our home that had gluten, dairy, or soy in it? Yeah, not my finest moment.

My husband wasn't thrilled about the fact that I had literally thrown away hundreds of dollars' worth of groceries. Then, the next day, after I went to the store to replace all the items I had trashed, he was even less enthusiastic when he saw that bill. Looking back now, it was not the way I would recommend anyone else go about this process.

A much better way to make the switch is to slowly replace one product at a time. (By the way, how are you doing with that list that's hanging on your refrigerator that you created in Chapter 3? Have you eaten through any of your food items and added them to the list of items to replace? Have you tried any new gluten-, dairy-, or soy-free products? Do you need any additional support? If so, scan this QR code and book a free call with my team to help you along the journey!)

Sadly, for many people who make the changes I am suggesting in this book, food costs will increase, even if you don't toss food like I did at the beginning of my journey. In this chapter, we're going to explore some of the reasons for this. It's important for you to understand that it might be more expensive to eat better. When we understand what obstacles are blocking our way, we can figure out how to overcome them. That's what this chapter is all about.

There's good news too. For some families, making this switch actually saves them money! It all depends on your family's habits beforehand and on how well you are able to implement some of the tips and tricks I'm going to share in this chapter. Healthy eating doesn't have to break the bank, and in this chapter we'll learn why.

Why It's Often (But Not Always) More Expensive to Eat Healthier

Bad "food" is cheap. We've probably all heard someone talk about how healthy food is more expensive to eat than junk food. In many ways, they are correct. Honestly, I don't even understand how some of the items we consume are considered food at all. They're not food. They're chemicals. Food is something found in nature, not something made in a lab.

Nonetheless, most of the "food" we eat in the U.S. is far removed from nature. This morning, as I was scrolling through some social media channels, I ran across a picture someone took of food they had purchased years ago from a fast-food restaurant. YEARS AGO. Not days. Not months. YEARS. This food wasn't moldy at all. It hadn't spoiled. In many ways, it looked exactly like it had when it was originally prepared. That's a problem. If the "food" we get from restaurants is so far removed from nature that mold won't even grow on it, that should make us rethink whether what we are consuming is actually food. It's not! Chemicals? Yes. Preservatives? Yes. Additives? Yes. But food? Many times, not so much.

Why is it that the food industry in this country favors processed foods so much more than fresh, healthy produce? In many ways, I think it all comes down to the mighty dollar.

Think of it this way. Which is more expensive to operate: a human being or a piece of equipment? Which is more dependable: a factory run on machines or a farm that depends on rain, sunlight, and a farmer? Equipment can be duplicated, improved, and made more efficient, but nature is unpredictable. People aren't machines, so they can't typically work as fast as machines can. Processed foods, because they are made by machines, are typically faster to produce and cost less in the long run than produce that is grown in the ground and farmed by real people.

There's also the issue of spoiling to consider. What is more cost-effective for a company: to sell a product that will last for months or to sell a product that will spoil in a week? Companies can create processed foods that don't go bad for months (sometimes even longer), so they can keep them on their shelves and not have to worry about losing profit because they spoil.

Go to any fast-food restaurant and look at the menu. Does it have a value section? If so, are there any healthy options on this part of the menu? Or is every "value" option unhealthy? Most value menus don't include salads or fresh fruits or vegetables. Rather, they include hamburgers, french fries, cheeseburgers, tater tots, and chicken nuggets (which don't have very much chicken in them at all—who are they trying to fool?). The healthier options are often higher in cost and are rarely included on value menus.

Because of these factors, it makes sense that it is more expensive for many families to eat healthier. Processed foods offer more calories for less money, thus giving consumers more "bang for their buck." If consumers want to save money, food manufacturers give them what they want in the form of processed junk "food."

But is it always more expensive to eat healthier than to eat the typical American diet? Many caregivers in my program do find their food expenses increase for the reasons we've just discussed, but there are also some families who see their food budgets shrink. Let's take a look at why this is sometimes the case.

Why Some Families SAVE Money When They Eat Healthier

Angela's eyes sparkled as she shared with me how much money her family was saving because of the dietary changes they had made. Her situation definitely wasn't the norm, so I was curious to learn more. "We used to eat out five or six times a week," she explained. "Now that I've started cooking more food at home, we are saving hundreds of dollars each week! I also used to buy pop for all of us. Cutting that out has saved us so much money!"

They ended up saving so much cash, in fact, that they planned a family vacation! Consider each of the following questions as they relate to your family's diet:

- Do you currently buy pop/soda?
- Do you drink fruit juice in your home?
- Do you buy large amounts of milk (not for cereal or baking, but just to drink)?

- Do your kids snack on cookies, chips, or similar products throughout the week?
- Do you currently eat out for many of your meals?
- When you eat out, do you order drinks?

If you answered yes to any of these questions, then you might find that making the changes I suggest in this book will actually save you money! Pop and fruit juice are unnecessary. So are large amounts of milk. As we discussed in an earlier chapter, drinking milk is not the only way to get the nutrients your body needs. Save your dairy-free milk for baking or for using in recipes. When thinking about what your child needs as far as liquids are concerned, stick with water or smoothies.

Another area to consider is snacking. If you buy a lot of processed snacks, especially if they are individually packaged, you might find that you will save a significant amount of money by removing these foods from your grocery list.

Finally, if you eat out regularly, and especially if you order drinks with each meal, you will likely save a significant amount of money by eating out less often, by not ordering drinks when you do eat out, and by cooking more from home. There are many benefits of cooking at home. Not only is it less expensive, as the markup in restaurants is huge, but it's also easier to control the ingredients and to guarantee your family is not accidentally consuming gluten, dairy, or soy. Eating from home is healthier and more affordable.

Eat Healthy Without Breaking the Bank: 14 Tips

Now that we've explored some of the possible reasons eating healthily might be more expensive (or less, depending on your current habits), let's look at some tips and tricks to help make eating healthy more affordable.

Money Saving Tip #1: Plan Your Meals

Meal planning is by far THE BEST thing families can do to save money on nutritious food. It prevents us from eating out at the last minute or grabbing convenience foods that cost more and aren't nutritious. Planning meals also enables us to group meals together that have common ingredients and to choose meals that make great leftovers. We can also make meals ahead of time with common ingredients and freeze them cooked or uncooked.

If you have never planned your meals ahead of time before, the best way to do this is to start slow. Plan one week at a time. Many families find it helpful to plan one week's meals and then repeat week to week. For instance, every week on Monday, a family might eat gluten-free pasta. Every week on Tuesday, they might eat tacos and so forth. By repeating week to week, it takes the stress out of meal planning and makes it super easy. If you're unsure how to plan meals, go back to Chapter 6 and read through it again for manageable steps and suggestions.

Money Saving Tip #2: Buy Food When It Is on Sale

I like to keep a running list of staples that my family will always eat. Then, when I see an item on this list go on sale, I stock up. By buying food when it's on sale, you save money in the long run.

Money Saving Tip #3: Don't Buy Everything Organic if You Can't Afford It

Many families assume they have to buy 100 percent organic produce. That's not the case. Of course, if you can afford all organic produce, that would be wonderful, but it's not an essential piece of a healthy diet. You can still have a nutritious diet without eating all organic produce. There are some foods that should always be purchased organic, but there are other foods that aren't as big of a deal. Take a look at the Dirty Dozen and Clean 15 lists that are published each year from the Environmental Working Group (https://www.ewg.org/) to figure out which produce to buy organic and which is okay to buy non-organic.

A food that's listed on the Dirty Dozen list is one you'll want to make sure to buy organic. Many families save money by exclusively buying the organic fruits and veggies that are on the Dirty Dozen list and buying "normal" produce for everything else. Don't feel bad doing this! It's a great compromise that keeps your family safe and healthy but also prevents you from wrecking your grocery budget.

Another tip to keep in mind is that sometimes local farmers may not be certified organic but nonetheless follow organic practices. You can feel secure buying from these farmers even though they don't technically have that organic label. Some questions to ask your local farmers include the following: 1) Do you use pesticides or fertilizers? 2) Do you use any genetically modified organism seeds? 3) Do you use any antibiotics or growth hormones? 4) How are your animals raised? How much exercise and open air do they get? 5) Is the food that the animals are being fed all organic?

Money Saving Tip #4: Buy Whole (Not Pre-Cut) Fruits and Vegetables in Season

Buy produce when it is in season. Have you ever noticed that produce prices vary significantly, based on the time of year you are buying them? That's because foods are more expensive when they are out of season and cheaper when in season.

Stock up when foods are in season and then freeze them for later. There are a few fruits and vegetables that don't freeze well (for instance, those with high water content), so if you're not sure, you can always search online to verify. Not only are you saving money by doing this, but you're also buying the foods when they offer the most nutritional value. By freezing them, you are locking in these nutrients and keeping your family healthy all year long. When buying fruit and veggies, also avoid the pre-cut varieties. They are more expensive.

Money Saving Tip #5: Stay Away from Processed Foods

Processed foods might be convenient, but they're also more expensive and not as nutritious. By limiting the number of processed foods purchased, many families are able to save significant amounts of money. When they do purchase processed foods (because let's be honest, it's not realistic for most families to NEVER buy them), they avoid individually wrapped products, choosing instead to buy larger packages and then separating them at home. Next time you buy raisins, nuts, trail mix, yogurt, chips, pretzels, and so on, avoid the individual boxes and opt instead for larger containers.

Money Saving Tip #6: Make Food from Scratch

Many foods can be made from scratch much more affordably than they can be purchased in a store. Consider the following products and whether you might be able to make these from scratch instead of buying in a store:

- Tomato/pasta sauce
- Gluten-free bread
- Pancake/waffle mixes
- Cookies
- Cakes

- Trail mix
- Taco seasoning
- Salad dressing

Gluten-free bread, in particular, is VERY EXPENSIVE, so I often suggest families not use it at all or make their own to save money.

Money Saving Tip #7: Buy Whole Chicken

Whole chicken gives the buyer more bang for their buck instead of buying chicken breasts, chicken thighs, and so on. When possible, choose to buy a whole chicken instead of separate parts. One other benefit of doing this is that the carcass and bones can then be used to make bone broth that can be used for future soups or other meals.

Money Saving Tip #8: Look for Discounted Meat

One of the ways that many families save a lot of money is by finding discounted meat and then freezing it straight away. Pay attention to when your local stores typically mark down their meat. Make it a practice to shop on these days so you have the opportunity to snag the cheapest meat possible.

Money Saving Tip #9: Have Meatless Mondays (or Tuesdays) or Buy Cheaper Proteins

Most likely, proteins will be your most expensive purchases at the grocery store. Cut down costs by having meatless meals once a week or by choosing cheaper proteins. Some inexpensive items that can be included in these meals are beans, lentils, quinoa, gluten-free oats, rice, and potatoes. Try buying dried beans instead of canned, and cooking and freezing them in smaller batches.

Money Saving Tip #10: Never Let Fruit Go to Waste

Freeze bananas or other fruit before they go bad to make homemade ice cream or use in smoothies. Don't assume that just because your bananas are a little black that they are no longer good! Just peel them and throw them into your freezer to use later on. We often use frozen bananas to create homemade ice cream.

Would you like to try some of my favorite homemade ice cream recipes? Gain access to them by scanning this QR code.

Money Saving Tip #11: Eat in Rather Than Out

Cooking at home, rather than eating out, is definitely the best way to both eat healthy and save money. It does involve meal planning but gets easier with time and practice.

Money Saving Tip #12: Plant a Garden

Planting a garden can significantly reduce the costs of buying fruit and vegetables in the store. Even if you don't want to go to the trouble of a large garden, you could still have some smaller herbs in your home in pots, along with a few potted vegetables. This is also a great way to get children involved. Many families find that their children who normally might refuse to eat a certain vegetable will eat it if they have grown it with their own hands! It's also a great way to teach children about what real food looks like.

Money Saving Tip #13: Shop with a List

The key to this tip is not only shopping with a list but also only buying items that are on the list. Don't allow yourself to give in to those impulse buys unless the item you see is one you actually need. Another tip that goes hand in hand with this one is to shop without your children if possible. Your children—if they are anything like mine—will ask you to buy items that aren't on your grocery list. If your kids aren't with you, they can't ask for things!

Money Saving Tip #14: Never Shop Hungry

One of the worst ways to shop is to shop hungry! That's because a hungry shopper will often give in to many more impulse buys, simply because everything looks delicious when they're hungry! Avoid shopping while hungry if at all possible.

Eating healthier does sometimes cost more. That is, unfortunately, the world we live in at the moment. My dream is that someday this will change, that someday our government will encourage healthy eating and encourage farmers who are producing safe, healthy produce and meat.

But we're not there yet. Until we get there, you and I have to choose. We can stay where we are—eating the same foods as the typical American—OR we can choose to live differently.

If you think about it, eating the typical American way is MORE expensive—not necessarily financially but in other ways. By eating poorly, the typical American is creating inflammation in their body. This inflammation, as we learned in chapters 1 and 2, can lead to challenging behaviors, mood issues, and a variety of health problems. The typical American might be spending less on groceries, but they are paying for it in other ways.

When children with ADHD are able to reduce the inflammation in their bodies, brains, and guts, their lives and behavior dramatically improve. The cost is worth the investment! Even if healthier food is more expensive for your family, keep in mind that though the food may cost a little more, it is a lifelong investment in better health! In the long run, when taking care of the body and feeding it the foods it needs, families save money on future medical bills, and they experience more happiness today.

What About Sneaking Food?

Another common obstacle many families face when trying to change their diets is a child who sneaks food. Even my own son does this from time to time, and we've been on this journey for years!

One of my team members told me the other day that when she began overhauling her family's diet, she couldn't figure out why her son's behavior wasn't improving. They didn't have any gluten or dairy in their house. None. She had tossed it all, so she was certain her son wasn't getting anything at home. She had also talked with her child's schoolteacher, so she didn't see how he could be getting anything at school either. She was baffled.

Then we ran a food sensitivity panel, and it showed that he was clearly eating gluten—and not just a little bit either! His results made it obvious that gluten was still a regular part of his diet. "How is this even possible?!" his mom asked me.

We investigated. We looked through her pantry for hidden sources of gluten. We checked her spices and seasoning packets. She even bought a new toaster because she thought maybe old breadcrumbs were the source of the gluten.

Finally, we found the culprit: the school cafeteria. Because school breakfasts and lunches were free at that time because of the pandemic, her son was sweet-talking the cafeteria workers (whom his mom had NOT spoken directly with) into giving him school meals. His teacher knew he wasn't supposed to be eating at the cafeteria, but the cafeteria staff did not. He was eating two breakfasts and two lunches each day: one that he brought from home and one that he grabbed at school. His poor mom couldn't believe it!

She assumed that because she didn't have gluten in the house, she was safe. She also assumed talking to her child's teacher would be enough. It wasn't. In the next couple of pages, I'm going to share some strategies that will help keep the sneaking food under control.

Sneaking Food Tip #1: Talk to EVERYONE

The mistake my team member made was that she didn't talk to everyone. She assumed that talking to her child's teacher would be enough to guarantee her child didn't eat anything at school. In a perfect world, this would work. That teacher would communicate with everyone else on the school staff, and there would be no opportunity for the child to eat anything without permission.

The reality, though, is that busy teachers are juggling multiple tasks each day. They are doing the best they can, but sometimes things get missed. It's a much safer option to speak with everyone at the school personally than to assume the message will be shared among staff.

Call or email the cafeteria staff, the school office, the librarian, the art teacher, the PE teacher, the music teacher, the counselor, the regular education teacher, any co-teachers, and anyone else you think might see your child at any point throughout the day. Many teachers give candy daily, and don't consider potential sensitivities outside of nuts. It is our job as our child's advocate to make sure to communicate with everyone who needs to know about their dietary changes.

One other thing to keep in mind, as far as school goes, is other students. Is it possible that other children will offer to share food with your child? It has happened MANY times in the families I work with: sometimes because other children don't know they shouldn't be sharing food and other times because they know the child isn't supposed to eat something and are helping them be sneaky! As you speak with the teacher, ask them to talk with the rest of the students about the importance of not sharing food with others because of potential allergies or sensitivities.

Along with the school, it's also important to communicate with family members, childcare providers, friends, and others who might be caring for your child on a regular basis. As discussed in the last chapter, you can make this easy on them by promising to provide the foods your child can have, so they don't have to worry about accidentally giving them something they shouldn't.

Sneaking Food Tip #2: Use Slip-Ups as Teachable Moments

There will be slip-ups. That's reality. The key is to take advantage of these slip-ups and use them as teachable moments. After a slip-up occurs, talk with your child about how their body felt after they sneaked the food and about how that food affected their behavior.

I like to check in with my children each night at dinner time and ask them how they have felt throughout the day. By making this a regular part of each day, it teaches our children to start to recognize their bodies and feelings.

Then, when they have a difficult day as a result of the food they ate, we can make the connection between their food and their feelings.

Eventually, as our children age, they will make their own food choices. By helping them connect the dots between their food and their feelings and behavior, we are helping them take ownership of the process. My son rarely sneaks food anymore, because he finally understands what it does to his body and how it affects his overall feelings of wellbeing. This wasn't an overnight success, though. It took MANY slip-ups and teachable moments for him to connect the dots. Remember, this is a process. The sneaking food, although not a fun thing to deal with, can sometimes be the best teacher of all, helping our children understand WHY we are doing what we're doing.

Sneaking Food Tip #3: Provide Plenty of Treats

If our children think the only way they will ever get a treat is to sneak it, they're going to sneak it. Part of being a child is enjoying special treats. Just because we are going gluten-, dairy-, and soy-free does NOT mean we can't have dessert!

Make sure you always have approved treats on hand. There are better-for-you alternatives to nearly every sweet treat! Your child should know that if they want a treat, they can get it—not by sneaking, but by asking.

Sneaking Food Tip #4: Get Your Child's Input

Another way to decrease the chances that your child will sneak food is to include them in the meal (and dessert) planning process. If children know what's coming up on the menu and they know they will enjoy the foods, they will be less likely to sneak foods that aren't on the menu.

Sneaking Food Tip #5: Get It Out of Your Home

The final way to curb sneaking food is to get the food out of your home. If the food isn't there, your child can't sneak it.

In my experience, the families who have the most success on this journey are those who participate as a whole family. It's not only the child who goes fully gluten-, dairy-, and soy-free but the entire family as well. This helps families be successful because it removes temptation. Far too often, children with whom I'm working don't improve because they are regularly sneaking gluten that is still in the home. The inflammation never has a chance to decrease because of the constant onslaught of gluten.

I know how difficult it can be to get the entire family on board. I also know that it's possible some people will never get on board, no matter how much you try to educate them on the damaging effects of gluten, dairy, and soy. They want to eat what they want to eat, no matter the consequences.

Are you familiar with Ron Swanson from the TV show *Parks and Recreation*? In this comedy show, Ron loves to eat high-fat foods that are terrible for him. He hates vegetables and refuses to make any healthy eating choices. In one episode, he gets sick and ends up having some lab work done, showing he has low potassium. As a nurse tries to convince him to eat more bananas, he says, "I live the way I live. I eat the things I eat. And I'll die the way I'll die."

If Ron sounds like someone in your home, then I would suggest having a designated spot for that person's foods that is locked away or out of reach of your child. Even if you can't convince your "Ron" to change their habits, you can still find ways to make their food inaccessible to your child.

Chapter Highlights

- One of the most common challenges families face when making the changes suggested in this book is the cost of eating healthier. Eating healthier is often more expensive than eating junk food, BUT there are things families can do to keep their healthy eating changes from devastating their bank accounts.

- Fourteen quick money-saving tips:
  - Tip 1: Plan your meals
  - Tip 2: Buy food when it is on sale
  - Tip 3: Don't buy everything organic if you can't afford it
  - Tip 4: Buy whole (not pre-cut) fruits and vegetables in season
  - Tip 5: Stay away from processed foods
  - Tip 6: Make food from scratch
  - Tip 7: Buy whole chicken
  - Tip 8: Look for discounted meat
  - Tip 9: Have meatless Mondays (or Tuesdays) or buy cheaper proteins
  - Tip 10: Never let fruit go to waste
  - Tip 11: Eat in rather than out
  - Tip 12: Plant a garden
  - Tip 13: Shop with a list
  - Tip 14: Never shop hungry

- When children with ADHD are able to reduce the inflammation in their bodies, brains, and guts, their lives and behavior dramatically improve, so even if healthier food is more expensive, the investment is worth it.

- Another common obstacle for many families is a child sneaking food. Here are some suggestions to help with this:
  - Talk to everyone who will be caring for your child about his or her dietary needs
  - Use slip-ups as teachable moments
  - Provide plenty of treats
  - Get your child's input
  - Get unapproved foods out of your home

Action Steps

1. How are you doing with the list that you created in Chapter 3 and that is hanging on your refrigerator? Have you eaten through any of your food items and added them to the list of items to replace? Have you tried any new gluten-, dairy-, or soy-free products? Do you need any additional help from my team? If so, scan the QR code at the end of this chapter to schedule a call with my team to discuss how we might be able to help you figure out your next steps on this journey.

2. Consider each of the following questions as they relate to your family's diet. If you answer YES to any of these questions, make the changes necessary to start saving money:
   - Do you currently buy pop/soda?
   - Do you drink fruit juice in your home?
   - Do you buy large amounts of milk (not for cereal or baking, but just to drink)?
   - Do your kids snack on cookies, chips, or similar products throughout the week?
   - Do you currently eat out for many of your meals?
   - When you eat out, do you order drinks?

3. Scan this QR code to gain access to the printable money-saving tips mentioned in this chapter or to grab your copy of our favorite homemade ice cream recipes.

4. Has your child sneaked any food recently? Think through the five tips mentioned in this chapter. Which one or several of these do you need to incorporate to help with this obstacle?

CHAPTER 11:

When Food Isn't Enough: The Missing Piece, Part 1

"Seriously, learn to control your child."

Those words haunted me for years. The woman who spoke them in the grocery store probably had no idea that her words would stick with me that long (or that I would be sharing them in this book years later). She was oblivious to the fact that I already felt like a failure as a parent. Her words cut me to my core—not because I didn't agree with her judgment but precisely because I did agree.

I thought I was a lousy mom too.

I had tried everything I could think of to "control" my child: medication, supplementation, essential oils, therapy, more discipline strategies than you can imagine, and so much more. Nothing did one bit of good.

Before I had a child with ADHD, I assumed—like this woman—that if caregivers were consistent, loving, and firm, then they could "control" a child.

That is what most of the parenting books say, after all. If parents do X, they get X result.

But what happens when parents do X and they don't get the anticipated result? What happens when a parent does X and the child responds with Y? Few of the parenting books I read when my son was little said anything about the possibility of a child not responding appropriately to a strategy.

I think that's because many parenting books are written with neurotypical children in mind. For neurotypical children, many of the traditional parenting methods are effective. When parents do X with a neurotypical child, they get X. The equation falls apart, however, with a neurodiverse child.

Caregivers cannot discipline their neurodiverse child in the same way they might discipline a neurotypical child. Deep down, I bet you already know this, though. My guess is, you've tried many parenting strategies that didn't work. You've probably already realized that traditional parenting methods don't work with children with ADHD. In the pages ahead, we're going to talk about some strategies that DO work.

You've already made a lot of changes, specifically in regard to the foods your family eats. In reality, though, changing the foods you eat isn't enough. I know, it's a big change, so it should be enough, right? I wish it were, but it's not. If caregivers only change the foods their children eat but continue to parent in ways that break down the relationship, the results will be miniscule. We also need to change the way we parent. That's because the most effective treatment considers the whole child. Not just the gut or the brain, but the entire person.

One of the problems with traditional medicine is that it takes the whole person out of the equation. It looks at individual symptoms and works to improve these. But it often fails to take into account how interconnected the body is. To see the best results, caregivers need to take the whole child into consideration, and that means thinking about the way we interact with them too.

In the pages ahead, I'm going to share some key concepts about parenting a child with ADHD. This is a HUGE topic, though, and certainly can't be covered in one chapter of a book. That's why my team and I asked a family and child therapist to help us create a fully online parenting course called ADHD Thrive Jumpstart 4 Parenting. Most parenting courses aren't designed specifically for children with ADHD. This course is. We realized that the only way to offer caregivers solutions that actually work with children with ADHD was to tailor the course for neurodiverse children. To learn more about this course, scan this QR code.

The Difference Between Punishment and Discipline

There's a significant difference between discipline and punishment. Award-winning author and social justice activist L.R. Knost explains it this way: "Discipline is helping a child solve a problem. Punishment is making a child suffer for having a problem." Discipline is all about teaching. Its purpose is to correct and inspire change.

Traditional parenting often confuses discipline with punishment. Traditional parenting says that if children do not obey, they should be punished. It assumes that this "punishment" will teach them to behave better. Punishment, though, doesn't teach. Or, if it does teach anything, it teaches a child to figure out a way to not get caught in the future.

Discipline, in contrast, focuses less on punishment and more on teaching. It focuses on re-dos when children practice doing what they should have done in the first place. It focuses on repairing relationships that might have gotten damaged through poor choices. It focuses on learning correct modes of behavior.

Don't misunderstand. With discipline, there are still consequences at times for negative actions. There are still boundaries and rules. But the focus is less on punishment when these rules get broken and more on teaching. Zig Ziglar, author and motivational speaker, defined it this way: "Punishment is what you do to someone; discipline is what you do for someone."

The general principles for positive discipline are listed here:

> **PRINCIPLES FOR POSITIVE DISCIPLINE:**
> 1. PRAISE GOOD BEHAVIOR.
> 2. SET EXPECTATIONS.
> 3. ADJUST YOUR MINDSET.
> 4. PICK YOUR BATTLES.
> 5. PROVIDE 1-ON-1 ATTENTION.
> 6. AVOID PUNISHMENT.

1. Praise Good Behavior

Children with ADHD receive significantly more negative messages throughout their lifetime than do children without ADHD. Some experts estimate they receive twenty thousand more negative messages by the age of ten.[61] Twenty thousand! That's a LOT of negativity!

It's not really all that surprising, though. Think about a typical day. How many everyday tasks are involved? While at home before school, there is brushing teeth, getting dressed, eating breakfast, packing a school lunch, getting shoes on, grabbing a coat, and getting to school on time. Then at school, there's a full day of sitting still, following instructions, staying in line, not talking out of turn, and the like. After school, there are chores, homework, nightly activities, and all of the tasks that are necessary to get to bed on time: brushing teeth again, showering, getting pajamas on, and so on.

ADHD isn't confined to one area of a child's life. It's not something they only have to deal with at school or in the mornings. Rather, it spans every single area of their lives, making many everyday tasks more challenging. Children with ADHD have to work so much harder than their neurotypical peers just to get through the day, so it's no wonder they often receive more negative feedback when they fall short.

As caregivers of children with ADHD, we have a significant opportunity to bridge the gap between the negative comments that a neurotypical child receives compared to the negative comments that a child with ADHD receives. We can help balance the scales.

Think of it like a cup. Every negative comment pokes a small hole in the cup, allowing our child's self-confidence to slowly leak out. When we pour in positive comments, we fill that cup back up. There will still be negative comments that continue to poke holes in their cup, but as long as we are consistently pouring in positive comments, we can make a huge impact. The way we respond to them, the way we parent them, the way we talk about their ADHD, the way we interact with them—all of that matters.

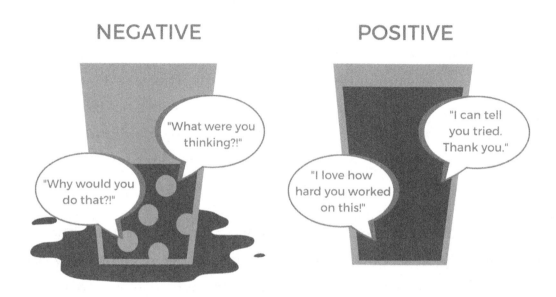

Through our interactions, we can either communicate to them that there is something wrong with them OR we can tell them they are uniquely made and have amazing gifts to offer the world. By catching them doing good things, we reinforce their positive self-confidence.

My absolute favorite way to do this is by using a "Caught You Doing Good" jar. In my kitchen, I have a glass jar. Beside the jar, I have a container full of tiny multicolored balls. Every time I "catch" my children doing good things, they get a ball in the jar. Once the jar is filled to the brim, we do something to celebrate. One night at dinner, my youngest son set a goal to earn 15 balls. He got us refills on our waters, took our trash to the receptacle, opened doors, and offered to help the entire family (even his brother, whom he rarely treats with kindness)!

2. Set Expectations

Children—especially children with ADHD—need to have clear expectations and boundaries. Boundaries help children feel safe and secure. They make their lives more predictable. It's critical for caregivers of children with ADHD to let their children know what is expected of them.

There are a few practical ways to do this. The first way is to sit down as a family and create family rules. Many families find it beneficial to write up their key family rules and post these rules somewhere in the home. Some possible rules to consider are: 1) We speak with kindness, 2) We use our hands and feet to help others, not to hurt them, 3) We use an inside voice, 4) We use our listening ears, and 5) We ask before touching someone else's belongings. Once the house rules are written, post them somewhere visible and refer to them often.

A second practical way to keep expectations in front of mind is to review them BEFORE going someplace where the boundaries might be difficult to maintain. For instance, when on a car ride to dinner, spell out for your children what you expect from them at the restaurant—for example, you expect them to use manners or try new foods or use an inside voice, and so on. By reviewing your expectations BEFORE going somewhere, you are setting your child up for success. It's much better to review the rules BEFORE than to remind them AFTER the damage has already been done.

A third practical way to set and keep expectations is to take advantage of routines. By building routines into your daily schedule, the routines begin to dictate a child's behavior, taking some of the pressure off you, the parent. It's the routine telling them what to do, rather than you as the parent. Children with ADHD often thrive under routines. In my experience, visual schedules tend to work very well with kids with ADHD. The visual schedules help them see and know exactly what comes next.

Keep in mind, though, that routines can take time to incorporate. Many caregivers start a routine and then quit when their children put up a fight. Not too long ago, one of the moms in my program came to me and said, "Dana, I've tried using an after-school routine with my son, but he fights it the entire time! I'm done trying!"

I understand her frustration. I have been there too. What I learned the hard way—and what I reminded her of—is that it takes time for a routine to stick. Don't throw in the towel just because it's not working after a couple of weeks. These routines aren't temporary. When they become a part of your life on a consistent basis, that's when they start really helping. Keep being consistent, even if it's hard during the first few weeks, and eventually you will start to see results.

There is one final caveat I want to add to this chapter. It's important that our expectations are realistically achievable for our kids. Many children with ADHD are actually several years behind in their emotional development. Though they might be ten years old chronologically, their emotional development might be more on par with a seven-year-old. As caregivers, we need to make sure our expectations are achievable. Otherwise, we will constantly be discouraged, and our kids will constantly fall short.

3. Adjust Your Mindset

Throughout this book, I've been sharing tips and tricks to help you make changes in your child. The truth of the matter, though, is that it's also critical for caregivers to make changes in themselves.

The most important change that needs to happen is a mindset shift. In the pages ahead, I'm going to share the top three mindset shifts caregivers need to make.

Mindset Shift #1: Our Children Are Doing the Best They Can

Shift your perception of your child from someone who is doing the wrong things BY CHOICE to someone who is still learning and who is doing their best. Everyone (your child included) wants to do well in life. No one wants to fight with those around them, feel uncontrollable big emotions, or constantly be in trouble. Your child doesn't want to exhibit the challenging behavior they are displaying; they simply don't have the skills necessary to handle whatever situation they are facing.

Best-selling author and child psychologist Dr. Ross Greene's famous mantra, "Kids do well when they can," became a constant companion for me when my son was really struggling with his ADHD symptoms. This mantra reminded me that my child wasn't intentionally wreaking havoc on our family. As the saying goes, he wasn't giving me a hard time. He was having a hard time.

This mindset shift doesn't make the problem behaviors disappear, but it does enable caregivers to handle those problems with more grace, empathy, and kindness toward their children.

Mindset Shift #2: Gratitude Isn't Optional

Parenting a child with ADHD is HARD—all caps HARD. From sunup to sundown, it brings with it challenges that threaten to destroy families. Marriages can easily be brought down by ADHD. So can sibling relationships, friendships, and other relationships within the family and wider community. ADHD is a devastating disorder because it affects every aspect of life.

Because of this, gratitude isn't a luxury for caregivers of children with ADHD. It's a necessity. About seven years ago, as I started down this ADHD journey with my oldest child, I began writing down a few things each day that I was thankful for, and the more I did it, the more I realized my attitude was changing. It wasn't that there were more things to be grateful for. Instead, it was that I NOTICED the things that were already there. I started looking for things to write in my journal, and this process helped me to find more and more blessings in my life.

On one especially difficult day, I remember sitting down to write in my journal and rethinking all of the events of the day. I started thinking about my son's rigid thinking. This kid would NOT take no for an answer and pushed and pushed and pushed if he didn't get his way. As I reflected on this challenge from a place of gratitude, I realized that this rigid thinking—this strong-willed behavior—was also a blessing. My son was persistent!

I had a choice that day: I could focus on his rigid thinking, or I could focus on his persistence. It was the same character quality, but a different way of looking at it. Practicing gratitude on a daily basis helped me change my perspective. It helped me make Mindset Shift #3 a reality. It enabled me to think things like, "My child isn't where I want him to be YET, but we are further along in this journey today than we were yesterday."

Gratitude doesn't always change our circumstances, but it DOES change the way we view them. As a parent of a child with ADHD, gratitude needs to be a consistent part of your daily routine.

Mindset Shift #3: ADHD Can Be a Gift (If You View It That Way)

When parenting a child with ADHD, it's sometimes difficult to look on the bright side. Thinking about the daily challenges ADHD presents—at home, at school, in just about every area of daily life—it's totally understandable that many caregivers forget about the benefits of ADHD. There are benefits, though. ADHD can be a gift *if* we learn to view it that way.

When my son's symptoms were at their worst, our entire family was miserable. It felt like we were on an emotional rollercoaster that wouldn't stop and that we couldn't ever get off of. There was hyperactivity. Impulsivity. Defiance. An inability to sit still. A lack of listening. The worst part of all was probably the emotional regulation challenges. Those meltdowns that seemed to happen on a daily basis were so hard at times. I understand why many caregivers struggle to see the glass as half full. ADHD can be really hard. That's precisely why it's critical for caregivers to remind themselves that ADHD isn't *only* a challenge; it's also a gift.

ADHD brings with it some really wonderful characteristics too. Think about the following characteristics that some people with ADHD possess. Remember, even if your child doesn't seem to excel in all of the following characteristics, they still have other amazing gifts and abilities. It's critical for caregivers of children with ADHD to focus on the child's strengths.

Persistence

Children with ADHD are some of the most persistent people I know. Granted, sometimes this looks like defiance. For instance, think about a child who won't put something down that they are working on when a parent tells them it's time to come to the table for dinner. This looks like defiance, but flip defiance on its side, and think about it differently. Defiance, when viewed through another lens, is persistence, and persistence is a wonderful thing! Challenges aren't going to stop a persistent person. Impossible isn't a word in their vocabulary. If they want something, they are going to do all they can to get it.

Creativity

There is a scientifically significant correlation between ADHD and creativity.[62] That means that people with ADHD have an advantage with creative activities! Think about singers Justin Timberlake and Adam Levine or celebrity host Ty Pennington. These famous men have been open about their struggles with ADHD. I can't help but wonder, though, if some of their success is also tied to their ADHD. Is it possible that their ADHD—though certainly challenging in some respects—also helped them become the people they are today? I think so.

Hyperfocus

Because of the words "attention deficit" in ADHD, some people mistakenly believe that those with ADHD can't focus on anything. That is absolutely not the case! A much better way to look at it, according to psychologist Kathleen Nadeau, is that those "with ADHD have a disregulated attention system."[63] It's hard for them to shift focus from something that interests them to something they find boring. Children with ADHD can actually hyperfocus on things they find interesting. Some children with ADHD can sit for hours working on one Lego masterpiece or art project. That kind of hyperfocus can be a huge benefit to them later on in life.

Passion

People with ADHD are passionate about things they love! Get them talking about a topic they are interested in, and it's very likely you'll learn A LOT about that subject matter! This passion is what led people like Olympic gymnast Simone Biles and Olympic swimmer Michael Phelps to push themselves and achieve greatness in their respective sports. These two athletes have both been open about their ADHD, but again, I wonder, did their ADHD also play a part in their success? Did their ADHD—and the passion that often accompanies it—help them become the athletes they are today?

Intelligence

Children with ADHD are often incredibly intelligent. They might not do well in school because of the challenges that traditional classrooms present for children with ADHD, but this isn't because of a lack of intelligence! In fact, many people with ADHD are actually gifted and show a lot of aptitude in certain subjects.

Think about someone with ADHD. My guess is that one or more of these characteristics describe them. One of the most important things we can do as caregivers of children with ADHD is to learn to focus on the positives of ADHD and to reframe the challenging characteristics. We do this by turning those negative attributes on their sides. It's not defiance; it's persistence. It's not ignoring; it's hyperfocus. By shifting the way we view ADHD, we can approach our children from a more positive framework.

4. Pick Your Battles

"My oldest child would do what he was told. Disobedience wasn't really an issue," Cassidy told me about her family dynamics as we discussed her youngest child with ADHD. "But then I had my second child, and he was totally different. Everything was a battle with him. Getting dressed in the morning. Brushing his teeth. Sitting at the table. Putting shoes on. Everything!"

Before Cassidy had her second child, she never really understood the importance of picking her battles. After all, you don't really have to pick your battles when there aren't battles to be had! After her second child with ADHD was born, though, that all changed, and she had a hands-on lesson on the importance of not sweating the small stuff.

As caregivers of children with ADHD, it's important for us to learn to pick our battles. I'm a Type A, hard-working, could-be-viewed-as-controlling type of mother. My personality, paired with my son's ADHD, could set us up for constant battles.

I decided a few years ago, though, that I didn't want my home to be a battleground. I don't want my children to look back on their time at home and only remember me barking orders at them. I want them to remember a happy childhood and a happy mother. In order for this to happen, I had to let go of some things and learn to pick my battles.

What are the nonnegotiables in your family? Make these the things you stand your ground on. As for everything else, let it go.

5. Provide One-on-One Attention

Spend at least 20 minutes each week giving each child in your home individual attention, doing an activity the child has chosen. Ideally, if you could spend time each day doing this, that would be best, but start with 20 minutes each week. This is critical to relationship building and trust. Children are much more likely to follow the instructions of a parent whom they feel close to. They might not listen simply because you're their parent, but they might because you've invested in them and have taken the time to build a strong relationship with them.

6. Avoid Punishment

Think back to the beginning of this chapter. Remember the difference between punishment and discipline? The goal here is DISCIPLINE because discipline is what really creates life change. Shift away from the mindset that your child needs to be constantly punished when making bad choices, and instead take opportunities for teachable moments.

When your child is displaying a behavior that is undesirable, try to remain calm and composed. Think of yourself as a coach, guiding your child toward success. Give them a specified time to alter what they are doing, expecting that initially they probably won't.

If the behavior continues after the allotted time is up, offer the child some thinking space. It is important that there not be negative connotations when asking your child to have some thinking space. Let them know it is not a punishment but a moment to calm down and reflect. Together with your child, find a place to go that is quiet. Initially you might need to sit with your child to show them how to effectively use the space. Your first priority here is getting the child to calm down.

Different techniques will work for different children. There is definitely not a one-size-fits-all model, but some strategies you could try include deep breathing techniques, mindful activities, fidgets, journals, coloring, calm down jars, and the like.

After the child has calmed down, you can then ask them to reflect on their behavior. A tool I have found useful for reflection is a thinking chart. In my home, the thinking chart is laminated and we use a whiteboard marker to check each box as we collect thoughts and ways to modify behavior. By using a laminated sheet, we are able to erase and use it again. Would you like a copy of the chart we use in my home? If so, scan this QR code to grab it.

Completing the thinking chart, whether written or spoken, is the child's passport to leaving the thinking area. Do not be disheartened if your child resists initially. Remember, change can take weeks. This is a marathon, not a sprint. Just as a child's inflammation cannot be reduced immediately, so also misbehaviors and unhealthy family patterns cannot be undone immediately either. It takes time, but I'm fully confident you can get there.

Chapter Highlights

- If caregivers change only the foods their children eat but continue to parent in ways that break down the relationship, the results will be miniscule.

- We also need to change the way we parent. That's because the most effective remedy considers the whole child—not just the gut or the brain, but the entire person.

- Traditional parenting often confuses discipline with punishment. Traditional parenting says that if a child does not listen, they should be punished and assumes "punishment" will teach them to behave better. Punishment doesn't teach. Discipline teaches.

- The key principles for positive parenting include the following:
  - Praise good behavior
  - Set expectations (through family rules, regular discussion of expectations, and routines)
  - Adjust your mindset:
    - Our children are doing the best they can
    - Gratitude isn't optional
    - ADHD can be a gift (if you view it that way)
  - Pick your battles
  - Provide one-on-one attention
  - Avoid punishment

Action Steps

1. We have joined forces with a Licensed Family and Child Therapist to put together a fully online parenting course called ADHD Thrive Jumpstart 4 Parenting. Most parenting courses aren't designed specifically for children with ADHD. This course is. We realized that the only way to offer caregivers solutions that actually work with children with ADHD was to tailor the course for neurodiverse children. To learn more about this course, scan this QR code.

2. After scanning the QR code, make sure and grab your copy of the Thinking Chart as well!

3. Looking over the six principles of positive parenting, which of these do you need to focus on most? You don't have to do everything today. Choose ONE of the strategies to put into practice this week.

4. Pick up a gratitude journal, if you don't already have one, and start practicing gratitude daily TODAY!

CHAPTER 12:

When Food Isn't Enough: The Missing Piece, Part 2

Jeff went through my program for his son who has ADHD and autism. He removed gluten, dairy, and soy completely from his child's diet. His son made improvements with the dietary changes—significant ones.

Before Jeff changed his son's diet, the child used to scream for hours on end. Once, Jeff timed him, and his screaming lasted for over two hours. He threw things at Jeff when he was out of control. If Jeff got too close to him during an "episode," he scratched, pinched, hit, or kicked him. He was eight when they began working with me. I still remember our original phone call. "I'm afraid he's going to really hurt me if we don't get this under control soon."

After three months of dietary changes, Jeff hopped onto another call with me. "He's doing better," he said. "He hasn't hurt me for over two months. His meltdowns are now more like five minutes instead of two hours. But he's still struggling. What am I doing wrong?"

Jeff wasn't doing anything wrong, and if that's where you find yourself too, you're probably not doing anything wrong either. I double-checked with Jeff that his son wasn't getting gluten from anywhere else. We walked through his activities. He checked in with the school to make sure he wasn't getting anything there. He also checked his pantry for any hidden sources of gluten. When we came up empty, I suggested he consider lab testing.

Sometimes, there is so much going on in the body of a child that changing the diet alone is not enough to fully reduce symptoms. Sometimes, it's necessary to go deeper. This chapter will dive into functional lab testing, explaining the "gold standard" tests used for children with ADHD and how these tests can help get to the bottom of what is really causing stress in the body. But first, let's look at when testing is necessary (and when it's not).

When Is Testing Necessary?

For about half the families I work with, testing isn't necessary. Once the diet is changed, symptoms subside enough that families don't feel the need to dive any deeper into underlying stressors. For families who have reached a place of calm and peace, there's no need to waste money on unnecessary tests. If they are happy, they are good to go!

On the other hand, for the other half of the families I work with, even after changing the diet, they still feel like something is missing. These families are the ones whom I recommend should move forward with functional lab testing.

I once had someone ask me if I'd ever worked with a child who showed no improvement after removing gluten, dairy, and soy. The answer to that is a firm no. Every single child I have worked with has shown at least some improvement by removing gluten, dairy, and soy and improving the diet. SOME improvement, though, isn't good enough for everyone.

Individual families have to decide for themselves what their end goal is. If changing the diet does not improve symptoms enough to make your family happy, that's when I recommend functional lab testing.

Functional lab testing allows us to look deep into the body, like with a microscope, to see what the underlying stressors are. Then, once we know what these stressors are, we are able to reduce them through targeted supplementation.

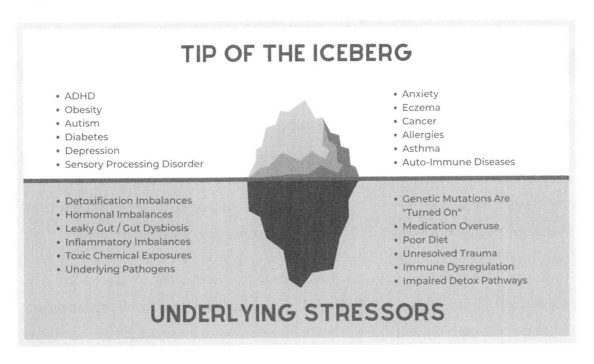

Take a look at the graphic above. In traditional medicine, most doctors treat symptoms or diseases. They treat ADHD, anxiety, asthma, allergies, and so on by treating the symptoms—the tip of the iceberg. If you have a cough, you get cough medicine. If you have a headache, you take a pain reliever. I'm not anti-medication. If I have a headache, I often take medication to get relief. Medication is not the problem; the methodology is the problem!

The problem is that this is a 100-percent cookie-cutter methodology. It's treating symptoms, not underlying stressors. It's not getting to the bottom of what's actually causing the cough or the headache. Take a look at the causes that fall below the water's surface. Wouldn't it be so much better for the person if we got to the underlying stressors instead of just the symptoms? Wouldn't it be so much better if we could, for instance, improve the poor diet that is to blame for the allergies, rather than just take allergy medication daily? I, for one, would much rather get to the bottom of what's causing a problem than put a bandage on it that's not doing anything for me long-term.

Another problem with this cookie-cutter methodology is that it's not looking at individual bodies, determining what these individual bodies need, and giving targeted treatment. It's treating every patient exactly the same, ignoring the fact that we are all individuals with unique genetic codes. My body is different from yours, so it likely needs different things than yours. When we treat every person exactly the same way and ignore what's underneath, we miss a huge opportunity to help someone long-term.

Functional lab testing gets to the underlying stressors in the body, the problems that are underneath. It's not just masking symptoms or slapping a bandage on a gaping wound but actually working to improve body functions. It's looking, as through a microscope, at the individual body. Take a look at what Amber told us after we ran functional lab tests on her daughter.

Amber
I have my daughter in Dana's program and it has been life changing. My daughter had been diagnosed with adhd, add, odd, and possible mthfr gene mutation and I was so tired of taking her to "specialists" who would put her on one medication from the next and nothing was working. Her behavior and hyperactivity were uncontrollable and no one had any answers and that is when I saw Dana's program on Facebook. Not one doctor or specialist ever mentioned anything about diet or functional lab testing. I decided it would be best to do both the nutrition program and lab testing because we were looking for more answers as to what was going on and Dana's program not only gave us the answers we had been looking for but she designed a program specifically for my daughter based on diet and supplements and it has been life changing. The hyperactivity, sleepless nights and behavioral outburst are gone. I wish I would have found Dana years ago.

Amber's daughter had multiple diagnoses and had seen numerous specialists before we met. She was hyperactive, oppositional, and regularly had behavior struggles. Functional lab testing gave us the answers we needed to help her. It told us what the underlying stressors were and allowed us to target these stressors with supplementation. For Amber and her family, testing was the way to go. It was the key that finally opened the door to transformation.

I don't know where you're sitting today as you read. Maybe you're still not fully gluten-, dairy-, or soy-free. That's okay! This is a journey. There's no need to rush. If this is where you find yourself, keep moving forward. Keep doing what you're doing. Every step forward is a step in the right direction. Put a bookmark in this chapter, and remember to come back to it once you've been fully gluten-, dairy-, and soy-free for a few months. Maybe by then you'll realize you don't need functional lab testing; that diet alone was enough to reduce your child's ADHD symptoms. Or maybe you'll realize testing would be beneficial for your family. Cross that bridge when you reach it.

If you're reading this chapter and your child with ADHD has been fully gluten-, dairy-, and soy-free for several months, then you have a decision to make. Are you where you want to be with your child's ADHD symptoms? Are you happy with the progress you've made? If so, feel free to skip over this last chapter. If not, stick with me. In the pages to come, I'm going to explain the four base tests I offer to families who want to dive deeper into the underlying stressors in their child's bodies.

Food Sensitivity Test

Do you remember in Chapter 1 when I explained leaky gut in detail? If you recall, I explained that leaky gut is when food particles slip through the intestinal walls and into the blood. The body views these food particles as foreign substances and creates an immune response to them, which can lead to a food sensitivity. I like to think of it like this: the body knows food isn't supposed to be in the blood, so when it sees it there, it attacks it. The more of that food a child eats, the more it leaks through the intestinal lining, and the stronger the immune response.

Before we dive into information about food sensitivity testing, though, it's important to understand the difference between allergies and sensitivities. There are different types of reactions to food. The three types we're going to look at are IgE, IgA, and IgG.

True food allergies (like those that require an EpiPen) are IgE reactions. These reactions are immediate (usually within an hour or so) and create noticeable effects like hives, trouble breathing, stomach upset, digestive issues, itchy mouth, and so on. IgE reactions can be mild or severe.

Food sensitivities, in contrast, are often delayed reactions and are thus harder to pinpoint. They are NOT life-threatening like true food allergies. IgA and IgG are both food sensitivity reactions and can cause symptoms like gastrointestinal issues, brain fog, skin rashes, hyperactivity, itching, and so on. Because food sensitivities (both IgA and IgG reactions) are harder to pinpoint, food sensitivity testing can be very beneficial.

IgE Reactions	IgA Reactions	IgG Reactions
True food allergy	*Food sensitivity*	*Food sensitivity*
Immediate reaction 1-3 days	*Delayed reaction 6-12 days*	*Delayed reaction an extended amount of time*
Symptoms range from mild to severe: hives, rash, inability to breathe, etc.	*Symptoms are typically gastrointestinal: stomach upset, gas, bloating, etc.*	*Symptoms vary widely as IgG responses can cause inflammation anywhere in the body.*

Food sensitivity testing looks at which foods in particular create those immune responses in the body. This is important information because the entire goal of making dietary changes is to reduce inflammation in the body. Those who have cut gluten, dairy, and soy from their diets have already taken huge steps toward reducing inflammation, but it's possible there are other foods creating inflammation too. That's what food sensitivity testing can tell us. Remember, inflammation leads to increased ADHD symptoms, so the more you can reduce inflammation, the quicker those symptoms can begin to decrease.

The trouble with food sensitivity testing, though, is that not all tests are created equal. Some of them are not very accurate, giving false positives or false negatives.

How do you know which test is best? In my experience, the best food sensitivity test is one that looks at food from the smallest peptide level. Stick with me for the next few paragraphs as I explain.

Think of food like a Lego masterpiece. My two children love to build with Legos. They build castles, cars, trucks, lighthouses, animals, and so many other amazing creations. Each of their masterpieces is composed of tons of different Legos; some blue, some red, some green, some large, some tiny. Think of food like a Lego masterpiece made of lots of individual pieces.

After you eat something, your body begins digesting the food. During digestion, the chewing and the stomach acid break down the food (your Lego masterpiece) into smaller and smaller chunks. By the time the food gets into your small intestine, it should, in theory, be broken down into individual Lego pieces.

Most food sensitivity testing uses bigger pieces called proteins to test and see if there's a reaction. I prefer to use food sensitivity tests that test down to the peptide level of the food. These tests are called *food zoomers*. Food zoomers get their name from the way they zoom in and test to see if there is a reaction on the peptide level.

Some foods are made up of thousands of peptides, just like a big Lego masterpiece could be made up of thousands of tiny unique Lego pieces. Zoomers are more precise, more comprehensive, and more definitive than other forms of food sensitivity testing, because a child may not be sensitive to the food protein (the large Lego piece) but could still be sensitive to a peptide that's part of that protein (the individual Lego piece used to build the larger Lego).

Once food sensitivity testing is complete, we know exactly which foods are causing inflammation in the body. We remove these foods temporarily (while continuing to avoid gluten, dairy, and soy also), give the body time to mend, and then hopefully reintroduce the sensitive foods after a period of time.

I created a functional lab testing video that explains the food sensitivity test I recommend, as well as other tests that are beneficial for children who need to delve deeper into what's causing stress in the body. If you'd like to watch this short video, you can do that by scanning this QR code.

Gut Test

Many families ask if they can ONLY do a food sensitivity test—and in the population of children we work with, there are always food sensitivities that show up. I understand the need to save money, but the gut isn't an area you want to skip. There is absolutely no point in doing food sensitivity testing if you're not also looking at other tests as well. That's because the food sensitivities are the direct result of something else that's going on in the gut. Something is CAUSING the food sensitivities. If that cause isn't dealt with, new food sensitivities are going to continue to pop up. You can remove one food, but another sensitivity will develop because you aren't fixing whatever caused the problem in the first place. This next test can help us determine the culprit behind the food sensitivities.

A stool test looks at the state of the gut overall. It looks for parasites, bacteria, worms, yeast overgrowth, and so on. It also looks at inflammation, immune system responses, leaky gut, reactivity to gluten, digestive enzymes, and how well someone is digesting fat.

Many times, this test is the KEY to unlocking a child's underlying stressors. Remember Jeff and his son? We ran several tests on him to see if we could figure out why he was still struggling. If we had only done the food sensitivity test, we would have removed peanuts, almonds, potatoes, corn, and eggs from his diet. That would have reduced inflammation because he was sensitive to these foods. It wouldn't, however, have dealt with the things that caused the sensitivities in the first place. Those things—four parasites! Jeff's son had four parasites that were wreaking havoc in his gut and creating so many problems for him. Without this test, we never would have known what was actually triggering the leaky gut and the food sensitivities.

Organic Acid Test

An organic acid test is also a really great test to run alongside the gut test and the food sensitivity test. The organic acid test (OAT for short) is a urine test that looks at important markers in the entire body.

It looks at potential nutrient deficiencies, diet modifications that might be necessary, detoxification pathways, neurotransmitters, yeast, mold, and so on. Basically, it looks at a whole host of complicated body systems and tells us what might be contributing to some of the symptoms in a child.

Kryptopyrrole Test

The final base test we run is called a kryptopyrrole test. Don't let that long word scare you. Pyrroles are a normal chemical byproduct in the body. They attach to vitamin B6 and zinc and draw these elements out of the body when they're excreted through the urine. If someone has elevated urine kryptopyrrole levels, it can result in a dramatic deficiency of zinc and vitamin B6. A high kryptopyrrole level can also be referred to as pyroluria, pyrrole disorder, or elevated pyrrole. It is often a contributing factor in behavior disorders, ADHD, depression, and assaultive, aggressive, and violent behavior.

Some of the symptoms common to pyroluria include the following.

- Poor tolerance to physical and emotional stress
- Irritability
- Anxiety
- Poor anger control
- Emotional mood swings
- Sensitivity to light or sound
- Poor short-term memory

Sometimes, when a family learns of elevated kryptopyrrole levels and then works to manage these levels through supplementation, they see dramatic improvements in behavior. The violence disappears. The emotional dysregulation settles. The anger subsides. This test is relatively inexpensive and can lead to amazing improvements, so it's one we regularly use with families who want to dive a little bit deeper with their child.

Summary

There you have it: the four base tests I recommend for families of children with ADHD who want to dive deeper into the possible underlying stressors in the body. There are other amazing tests that are great for families to do after these four base tests are complete, but I prefer to begin with these. Using these four tests, I like to see what kind of progress we can make. I'd rather the families I work with not spend more money than necessary, so if we can get where we need to go with these four tests alone, that's where I like to start.

It's certainly possible to do more than these four tests, and, of course, doing more tests will provide more information. However, there are only so many issues a caregiver can tackle at once. Why not start here and save money by not doing all the tests that are available and only dive further if absolutely required?

Maybe you read this chapter and realized this is what you need to do for your family. You've changed the diet. Now you need to dive deeper. If this is you, scan the QR code in the Action Steps and book a call with my team to further discuss lab testing and what that looks like.

Chapter Highlights

- Sometimes, a family can remove gluten, dairy, and soy, replace these foods with healthy alternatives, and still not see the full reduction in symptoms they wished to see. In these cases, it may be necessary to do functional lab testing.

- Functional lab testing allows us to dive deeper into the underlying stressors in the body. It enables us to find those stressors and then reduce them through targeted supplementation.

- The following tests are the ones I recommend first:
  - Food sensitivity test (down to the peptide level), a blood test
  - Gut test, a stool test
  - Organic acid test, a urine test
  - Kryptopyrrole test, a urine test

Action Steps

1. Think about the progress you have made. Answer the following questions for yourself:
   - Are you fully gluten-, dairy-, and soy-free? If not, what steps do you need to take to get there in the weeks to come?
   - If you are fully gluten-, dairy-, and soy-free, have you seen the progress you wanted to see? If so, take some time to celebrate your success! If not, do you think functional lab testing would be beneficial for your child?

2. Scan this QR code to watch that training video about lab testing or to book a free call with my team to discuss it in depth.

Conclusion

"How long is it going to take before I start seeing significant improvements?"

It's one of the most common questions I get asked. Believe me, I get it. Caregivers of children with ADHD are often desperate for solutions. They are miserable because of the out-of-control behavior of their children. They might have tried medication. Or supplements. Or essential oils. Or parenting strategies. Or therapy. Or all of the above. They have likely done everything they can think of to do. Maybe that's why you chose to pick up this book. Maybe you were feeling desperate too.

I wish I could make a promise with a timetable: *If you do the things in this book, your child's ADHD symptoms will completely disappear within two months.* Wouldn't that be nice? Unfortunately, every child is so different. Everyone's body is different. Every family is different. I can't promise you the ADHD symptoms will completely disappear in two months. I can't promise you they'll disappear at all.

What I can promise you is that no matter what, the changes I'm suggesting in this book will help your child and your family. They will improve your health, your emotional well-being, and your happiness. They might not fix everything, but they will make a difference in a positive way.

I don't want this chapter to be goodbye. I would love to stay in touch with you and help you as you continue this journey. As I've said before, this isn't a quick fix. It's a life change. I would be honored to continue to be a part of that change in the years to come. If you'd like to continue to learn more about natural solutions for ADHD, you can join my mailing list by scanning the following QR code. That QR code will also give you access to all of the bonus material that I've mentioned throughout this book. I hope these bonuses help you on your journey. If you're unable to scan this QR code, you can find all the bonus resources at this link:

https://programs.adhdthriveinstitute.com/offers/G2xFNwTK/checkout

Finally, I want to invite you to leave a book review. Other caregivers of children with ADHD need to know they have options. They need to know that if they don't want to try medication, there are alternatives that are effective. Your book review will let the Amazon algorithms know this book is worth reading. It will tell Amazon this book is worth suggesting to other caregivers who are searching for answers. You can be a part of the solution just by leaving a review.

Thank you for going on this journey with me.

Glossary

ADHD (attention deficit hyperactivity disorder): a neurodevelopmental condition characterized by inattention, hyperactivity, and impulsiveness

Azodicarbonamide: a chemical additive used as a whitening agent in cereals and breads in the United States but banned by the European Union

Bacillus thuringiensis (Bt) eggplant: an eggplant that has been genetically modified, the first GMO in South Asia

Bromate: potassium bromate is a food additive often used in bread that is banned in other countries but allowed in the United States

Brominated vegetable oil (BVO): a food additive used in the United States in many citrus soft drinks but banned by the European Union—interestingly enough, BVO is also a flame retardant for plastics

Candida: yeast, a type of fungus that, when overgrown, can cause diseases in the body

Carbohydrates: also known as carbs, carbohydrates are a type of nutrient found in food—contrary to popular belief, not all carbohydrates are bad; in fact, carbohydrates, along with protein and fat, are necessary for our bodies to thrive

Carcinogen: a substance that might cause cancer in humans

Casein: the main protein found in milk

Casomorphin: an opioid peptide that is produced as the body digests milk products

Choline: an important nutrient that is found in eggs and other foods

Coumarin: a chemical compound naturally occurring in cinnamon that is dangerous if consumed in large quantities—cassia cinnamon has higher amounts of coumarin than Ceylon cinnamon; therefore, Ceylon cinnamon is preferred

Detoxification pathways: the way in which our bodies eliminate toxins and things they don't need

Dopamine: a neurotransmitter that is responsible for how we feel pleasure and helps the body balance mood and regulate emotion

Endocrine disruptor: a compound that disrupts or interferes with the endocrine system, the messenger system that distributes hormones throughout the body

Enzyme: proteins that speed up reactions in the body; digestive enzymes help break down food in the body

Frontal lobe: the front part of the brain, responsible for a variety of bodily functions, such as memory, emotions, impulse control, attention, and so on

Glutamate: an amino acid that can be found naturally in the body and in food but also can be created in a lab; high levels of glutamate can be problematic

Gluteomorphins: an opioid peptide that is developed as the body digests gluten

GMOs (genetically modified organisms): living organisms that have been changed on a genetic level—the appealing gene in the original organism is noted, copied, and inserted into another organism, the GMO

Gut-brain connection: the communication between the gut and the brain

Gut dysbiosis: the state of imbalance in gut bacteria

Gut microorganisms: microorganisms (like bacteria) that live in the digestive system

Herbicide: commonly called weedkiller, a herbicide is a substance that is used to kill unwanted plants

H. pylori: a type of bacteria that can cause infection or inflammation in the upper GI tract, short for *Helicobacter pylori*

IgA (immunoglobulin A): an antibody responsible for a type of delayed immune reaction to food, typically within 6 to 12 days and often gastrointestinal

IgE (immunoglobulin E): an antibody responsible for a true allergic reaction to food that occurs immediately or shortly thereafter; symptoms can range from mild to severe

IgG (immunoglobulin G): an antibody responsible for a delayed immune reaction to food that can occur over an extended amount of time; symptoms can vary widely

Immunological response: the way in which the body defends itself against a threat or perceived threat

Inflammation: the body's natural reaction to an irritant

Insecticide: a substance used to kill insects

Isoflavones: plant-based estrogens, found in soy

Leaky gut: a condition that results from increased intestinal permeability, whereby food particles slip through the intestinal walls and into the bloodstream

Micronutrients: vitamins and minerals that are essential for a healthy body

Microorganisms: microscopic organisms, such as bacteria

MSG (monosodium glutamate): a food additive derived from glutamic acid and used to enhance the flavor in some foods

Neuro-behavioral disorders: disorders that are primarily associated with the brain

Neurotransmitters: the chemical messengers of the body, responsible for sending signals throughout the body

Olestra: a fat substitute that is banned in many countries but allowed in food in the United States

Oligomeric proanthocyanidins: a plant-derived compound that fights against environmental toxins; can be used as an herbal supplement

Permeability: the quality of an item (in this book, the lining of the gut) that determines how well particles pass through it

Pesticide: a substance that is used to prevent pests, such as insects or weeds, that might harm plants or animals; herbicides and insecticides are two types of pesticides

Phytonutrients: nutrients found in certain plants and superfoods that are beneficial for the body

Potassium bromate: *see* bromate

Pyroluria: pyrrole disorder, a condition that can lower key vitamins and minerals in the body

Red 40: an artificial food coloring made from petroleum, banned by some countries, requiring a warning label by others, but allowed in the United States; linked to adverse effects in children

Serotonin: a neurotransmitter that helps the body balance mood and regulate emotion

SSRIs (selective serotonin reuptake inhibitors): a class of drugs typically used to treat depression

Theobromine: a molecule found in plants, especially cacao, that has many health benefits

Vagus nerve: carries signals between the digestive system and the brain and vice versa

Yellow 5: an artificial food coloring made from petroleum, banned by some countries, requiring a warning label by others, but allowed in the United States; linked to adverse effects in children

Yellow 6: an artificial food coloring made from petroleum, banned by some countries, requiring a warning label by others, but allowed in the United States; linked to adverse effects in children

Code Words for Sugar

- Corn sweetener
- Corn syrup
- Corn syrup solids
- Dehydrated cane juice
- Dextrin
- Dextrose
- Glucose
- Lactose
- Maltodextrin
- Maltose
- Malt syrup
- Molasses
- Rice syrup
- Saccharose
- Sorghum or sorghum syrup
- Sucrose
- Xylose

Code Words for Gluten

- Artificial flavors and colors (may contain gluten)
- Barley
- Bran
- Bulgur
- Citric acid (may contain gluten)
- Couscous
- Dextrin/maltodextrin (may contain gluten)
- Durum
- Einkorn
- Emmer
- Farina
- Flour, unless certified gluten-free (this includes white flour, bread flour, wheat flour, all-purpose flour, etc.—unless it is labeled gluten-free, you can assume it contains gluten)
- Kamut
- Malt
- Modified starch/modified food starch (can contain gluten)
- Monosodium glutamate (MSG), may contain gluten
- Natural flavors (sometimes these are made from gluten-containing ingredients)
- Oats should be certified gluten-free—otherwise, assume they are contaminated with gluten
- Rye
- Seasonings—some may contain gluten
- Seitan
- Semolina
- Spelt

- Triticale
- Vegetable protein/hydrolyzed vegetable protein (may contain gluten)
- Wheat
- Yeast extract, may contain gluten (note: though yeast is naturally gluten-free, yeast extract is often NOT; if you are unsure, look for the certified gluten-free label)

Code Words for Dairy

- Artificial butter
- Artificial flavors (may contain dairy)
- Butter
- Caramel flavoring (may contain dairy)
- Casein
- Caseinates
- Cheese
- Cheese flavor
- Chocolate (may contain dairy)
- Cream
- Curd
- Custard
- Diacetyl
- Goat's milk
- Half and half
- Hydrolysates
- Ice cream
- Kefir
- Lactose

- Milk (this includes all types of milk, even lactose-free milk, unless labeled dairy-free)
- Natural flavors (may contain dairy)
- Nougat
- Paneer
- Pudding
- Sherbet
- Whey
- Yogurt

Endnotes

1. McQueen, Janie. "All the Facts and Stats on ADHD in One Page." *WebMD*, https://www.webmd.com/add-adhd/adhd-facts-statistics. Medically Reviewed by Smitha Bhandari, MD on 02 July 2020. Accessed 06 Jan. 2022.

2. Visser, Susanna N., et al. "Trends in the Parent—Report of Health Care Provider—Diagnosed and Medicated Attention-Deficit/Hyperactivity Disorder: United States, 2003–2011." *Journal of the American Academy of Child and Adolescent Psychiatry*, U.S. National Library of Medicine, Jan. 2014, https://www.ncbi.nlm.nih.gov/pmc/articles/PMC4473855/. Accessed 06 Jan. 2022.

3. This book is not intended as a substitute for the medical advice of physicians. The reader should consult a physician in matters relating to health and particularly with respect to symptoms that may require diagnosis or medical attention.

4. Buckley, Aaron, and Jerrold R. Turner. "Cell Biology of Tight Junction Barrier Regulation and Mucosal Disease." *Cold Spring Harbor Perspectives in Biology*, Cold Spring Harbor Laboratory Press, 02 Jan. 2018, https://www.ncbi.nlm.nih.gov/pmc/articles/PMC5749156/. Accessed 02 Feb. 2022.

5. Pelsser, Dr. Lidy M., et al. "Effects of a Restricted Elimination Diet on the Behaviour of Children with Attention-Deficit Hyperactivity Disorder (INCA Study): A Randomised Controlled Trial." *The Lancet*, 05 Feb. 2011, https://www.thelancet.com/journals/lancet/article/PIIS0140-6736(10)62227-1/fulltext. Accessed 06 Jan. 2022.

6. "ADHD (Attention Deficit and Hyperactivity Disorder)." *Food for the Brain*, 09 Nov. 2020, https://foodforthebrain.org/condition/adhd-and-hyperactivity/. Accessed 06 Jan. 2022.

7. Parker, Gordon, and Tim Watkins. "Treatment-Resistant Depression: When Antidepressant Drug Intolerance May Indicate Food Intolerance." *The Australian and New Zealand Journal of Psychiatry*, U.S. National Library of Medicine, Apr. 2002, https://pubmed.ncbi.nlm.nih.gov/11982551/. Accessed 06 Jan. 2022.

8. Schwartz, D. L., Gilstad-Hayden, K., Carroll-Scott, A., Grilo, S. A., McCaslin, C., Schwartz, M., Ickovics, J. R., "Energy Drinks and Youth Self-Reported Hyperactivity/Inattention Symptoms." *Academic Pediatrics*, U.S. National Library of Medicine, 09 Feb. 2015, https://pubmed.ncbi.nlm.nih.gov/25676784/. Accessed 07 Jan. 2022.

9. Rucklidge, J. J., Eggleston, M. J. F., Johnstone, J. M., Darling, K., Frampton, C. M., "Vitamin-Mineral Treatment Improves Aggression and Emotional Regulation in Children with ADHD: A Fully Blinded, Randomized, Placebo-Controlled Trial." *Journal of Child Psychology and Psychiatry, and Allied Disciplines*, U.S. National Library of Medicine, 02 Oct. 2017, https://pubmed.ncbi.nlm.nih.gov/28967099/. Accessed 07 Jan. 2022.

10. "Parent Ratings of Behavioral Effects of Biomedical Interventions." Autism Research Institute, Mar. 2009, https://www.autism.org/treatment-ratings-for-autism/ and https://www.autism.org/wp-content/uploads/2018/12/ParentRatings2009.pdf. Accessed 07 Jan. 2022.

11. Sanchez, Bianca. "These 16 Things in US Food Are Banned in Other Countries." *The Daily Meal*, The Daily Meal, 01 July 2020, https://www.thedailymeal.com/travel/american-foods-banned-other-countries.

12. Hollon, J., Puppa, E. L., Greenwald, B., Goldberg, E., Guerrerio, A., Fasano, A., "Effect of Gliadin on Permeability of Intestinal Biopsy Explants from Celiac Disease Patients and Patients with Non-Celiac Gluten Sensitivity." *Nutrients*, U.S. National Library of Medicine, 27 Feb. 2015, https://pubmed.ncbi.nlm.nih.gov/25734566/. Accessed 07 Jan. 2022.

13. Bell, Becky. "Is Leaky Gut Syndrome a Real Condition? An Unbiased Look." *Healthline*, Healthline Media, 02 Feb. 2017, https://www.healthline.com/nutrition/is-leaky-gut-real#TOC_TITLE_HDR_2. Accessed 07 Jan. 2022.

14. Unfortunately, even though there is significant evidence supporting the understanding of leaky gut, mainstream medical professionals sometimes deny its existence. Because of this, leaky gut alone is not a diagnosable condition. Medical professionals do, however, agree that increased intestinal permeability is a problem that can lead to chronic conditions.

15. Nett, Amy. "Glutamate—Could Its Hidden Sources Be Harming Your Health?" *Chris Kresser*, 16 Sept. 2014, https://chriskresser.com/beyond-msg-could-hidden-sources-of-glutamate-be-harming-your-health/. Accessed 07 Jan. 2022.

16. "Definition & Facts for Lactose Intolerance." *National Institute of Diabetes and Digestive and Kidney Diseases*, U.S. Department of Health and Human Services, https://www.niddk.nih.gov/health-information/digestive-diseases/lactose-intolerance/definition-facts. Accessed 07 Jan. 2022.

17. Prinz, Robert, et al. "Dietary Correlates of Hyperactive Behavior in Children." *Journal of Consulting and Clinical Psychology*, vol. 48, no. 6, 1980, pp. 760–769. As cited by editors, *ADDitude*. "Why Sugar Is Kryptonite: ADHD Diet Truths." *ADDitude*, 19 July 2021, https://www.additudemag.com/adhd-diet-nutrition-sugar/. Accessed 07 Jan. 2022.

18. Yu, C.-J., Du, J.-C., Chiou, H.-C., Feng, C.-C., Chung, M.-Y., Yang, W., Chen, Y.-S., Chien, L.-C., Hwang, B., Chen, M.-L., "Sugar-Sweetened Beverage Consumption Is Adversely Associated with Childhood Attention Deficit/Hyperactivity Disorder." *International Journal of Environmental Research and Public Health*, U.S. National Library of Medicine, 04 July 2016, https://pubmed.ncbi.nlm.nih.gov/27384573/. Accessed 02 Feb. 2022.

19. Johnson, Richard J., et al. "Attention-Deficit/Hyperactivity Disorder: Is it Time to Reappraise the Role of Sugar Consumption?" Sept. 2011, https://www.ncbi.nlm.nih.gov/pmc/articles/PMC3598008/. Accessed 02 Feb. 2022.

20. Stevens, Laura, M.Sci. "Feed Your Child's Focus: ADHD Foods, Dyes & Attention." *ADDitude*, ADDitude, 08 Apr. 2021, https://www.additudemag.com/feed-your-childs-focus-adhd-food-nutrition/. Accessed 12 Oct. 2021.

21. For a longer list of flour alternatives, check out the following: Goodson, Amy. "The 14 Best Gluten-Free Flours." *Healthline, Healthline* Media, 30 May 2018, https://www.healthline.com/nutrition/gluten-free-flours#section3. Accessed 07 Jan. 2022.

22. Lara S. Ford, MD, MPH, Steve L. Taylor, PhD, Robert Pacenza, BA, Lynn M. Niemann, Debra M. Lambrecht, BS, Scott H. Sicherer, MD. "Food Allergen Advisory Labeling and Product Contamination with Egg, Milk, and Peanut." *The Journal of Allergy and Clinical Immunology*, 12 July 2010, https://www.jacionline.org/article/S0091-6749(10)00891-2/fulltext. Accessed 02 Feb. 2022.

23. "Water: Essential to Your Body." *Mayo Clinic Health System*, 22 July 2020, https://www.mayoclinichealthsystem.org/hometown-health/speaking-of-health/water-essential-to-your-body. Accessed 28 Oct. 2021.

24. Rethy, Janine. "Choose Water for Healthy Hydration." *HealthyChildren.org*, 27 Jan. 2020, https://www.healthychildren.org/English/healthy-living/nutrition/Pages/Choose-Water-for-Healthy-Hydration.aspx. Accessed 28 Oct. 2021.

25. Kianoush, S., Balali-Mood, M., Mousavi, S. R., Moradi, V., Sadeghi, M., Dadpour, B., Rajabi, O., Shakeri, M. T., "Comparison of Therapeutic Effects of Garlic and D-Penicillamine in Patients with Chronic Occupational Lead Poisoning." *Basic & Clinical Pharmacology & Toxicology*, U.S. National Library of Medicine, 29 Dec. 2011, https://pubmed.ncbi.nlm.nih.gov/22151785/. Accessed 02 Nov. 2021.

26. Cai, Huizhen, et al. "Practical Application of Antidiabetic Efficacy of Lycium Barbarum Polysaccharide in Patients with Type 2 Diabetes." *Medicinal Chemistry (Shariqah (United Arab Emirates))*, Bentham Science Publishers, June 2015, https://www.ncbi.nlm.nih.gov/pmc/articles/PMC4475782/. Accessed 02 Nov. 2021.

27. Nance, Dwight M., and Harunobu Amagase. "A Randomized, Double-Blind, Placebo-Controlled, Clinical Study of the General Effects of a Standardized Lycium Barbarum (GOJI) Juice, GoChi." *Journal of Alternative and Complementary Medicine (New York, N.Y.)*, U.S. National Library of Medicine, 14 May 2008, https://pubmed.ncbi.nlm.nih.gov/18447631/. Accessed 02 Nov. 2021.

28. For a detailed timeline and more information about GMOs, visit the following website: Center for Food Safety and Applied Nutrition. "Science and History of GMOs and Other Food Modification Processes." *U.S. Food and Drug Administration*, FDA, https://www.fda.gov/food/agricultural-biotechnology/science-and-history-gmos-and-other-food-modification-processes. Accessed 10 Jan. 2022.

29. Gashler, Krisy. "BT Eggplant Improving Lives in Bangladesh." *Cornell Chronicle*, 16 July 2018, https://news.cornell.edu/stories/2018/07/bt-eggplant-improving-lives-bangladesh. Accessed 09 Nov. 2021.

30. Hsaio, Jennifer. "GMOs and Pesticides: Helpful or Harmful?" *Science in the News*, 10 Aug. 2015, https://sitn.hms.harvard.edu/flash/2015/gmos-and-pesticides/. Accessed 09 Nov. 2021.

31. Cressey, Daniel. "Widely Used Herbicide Linked to Cancer." *Scientific American*, Scientific American, 25 Mar. 2015, https://www.scientificamerican.com/article/widely-used-herbicide-linked-to-cancer/. Accessed 09 Nov. 2021.

32. Séralini, Gilles-Eric, et al. "Republished Study: Long-Term Toxicity of a Roundup Herbicide and a Roundup-Tolerant Genetically Modified Maize." *Environmental Sciences Europe*, Springer Berlin Heidelberg, 24 June 2014, https://www.ncbi.nlm.nih.gov/pmc/articles/PMC5044955/. Accessed 02 Feb. 2022.

33. For more information about GMO labeling, check out the following website: https://www.centerforfoodsafety.org/issues/976/ge-food-labeling/international-labeling-laws. Accessed 02 Feb. 2022.

34. NonGMO Project. "Americans Deserve Better Than the USDA's GMO Labeling Law." *Non-GMO Project*, https://www.nongmoproject.org/blog/americans-deserve-better-than-the-usdas-gmo-labeling-law/. Accessed 09 Nov. 2021.

35. "List of Bioengineered Foods." *List of Bioengineered Foods | Agricultural Marketing Service*, https://www.ams.usda.gov/rules-regulations/be/bioengineered-foods-list. Accessed 09 Nov. 2021.

36. Center for Food Safety and Applied Nutrition. "GMO Crops, Animal Food, and Beyond." *U.S. Food and Drug Administration*, FDA, https://www.fda.gov/food/agricultural-biotechnology/gmo-crops-animal-food-and-beyond. Accessed 09 Nov. 2021.

37. Nancy L. Swanson, Andre Leu, Jon Abrahamson, & Bradley Wallet. "Genetically Engineered Crops, Glyphosate and the Deterioration of Health in the United States of America." *Journal of Organic Systems*, 2014, https://www.organic-systems.org/journal/92/JOS_Volume-9_Number-2_Nov_2014-Swanson-et-al.pdf. Accessed 04 Feb. 2022.

38. Nancy L. Swanson, Andre Leu, Jon Abrahamson, & Bradley Wallet. "Genetically Engineered Crops, Glyphosate and the Deterioration of Health in the United States of America." *Journal of Organic Systems*, 2014, https://www.organic-systems.org/journal/92/JOS_Volume-9_Number-2_Nov_2014-Swanson-et-al.pdf. Accessed 04 Feb. 2022.

39. Amy Dean, D.O., and Jennifer Armstrong, M.D. "Genetically Modified Foods." *American Academy of Environmental Medicine*, 8 May 2009, https://www.aaemonline.org/genetically-modified-foods/. Accessed 02 Feb. 2022.

40. Center for Food Safety and Applied Nutrition. "GMO Crops, Animal Food, and Beyond." *U.S. Food and Drug Administration*, FDA, https://www.fda.gov/food/agricultural-biotechnology/gmo-crops-animal-food-and-beyond. Accessed 09 Nov. 2021.

41. "GMO Facts." *Non-GMO Project*, https://www.nongmoproject.org/gmo-facts/. Accessed 12 Nov. 2021.

42. Duke, S. O., and Powles, S. B. (2009). "Glyphosate-resistant crops and weeds: Now and in the future." *AgBioForum*, 12(3&4), 346–357.

43. "Organic Practices Factsheet." *Agricultural Marketing Service*. https://www.ams.usda.gov/publications/content/introduction-organic-practices. Accessed 15, April. 2022.

44. "How to Spot Those Sneaky Sources of Gluten." *Cleveland Clinic*, 23 Mar. 2021, https://health.clevelandclinic.org/spot-secret-sources-gluten-infographic/. Accessed 30 Dec. 2021.

45. "How to Spot Those Sneaky Sources of Gluten." *Cleveland Clinic*, 23 Mar. 2021, https://health.clevelandclinic.org/spot-secret-sources-gluten-infographic/. Accessed 30 Dec. 2021.

46. This book is not intended as a substitute for the medical advice of physicians. The reader should consult a physician in matters relating to health and particularly with respect to symptoms that may require diagnosis or medical attention.

47. Walle, Gavin Van De. "Polyunsaturated Fat: Definition, Foods, Benefits and Risks." *Healthline*, Healthline Media, 31 Oct. 2018, https://www.healthline.com/nutrition/polyunsaturated-fat#risks. Accessed 23 Nov. 2021.

48. Hallowell, Edward, et al. "Can a Daily Fish Oil Supplement Help Curb Symptoms of ADHD?" *ADDitude*, ADDitude, Updated 05 Jan. 2022, https://www.additudemag.com/fish-oil-for-adhd-symptoms/. Accessed 23 Nov. 2021.

49. LaChance, Laura, et al. "Omega-6 to Omega-3 Fatty Acid Ratio in Patients with ADHD: A Meta-Analysis." *Journal of the Canadian Academy of Child and Adolescent Psychiatry = Journal de l'Académie Canadienne de Psychiatrie de l'Enfant et de l'Adolescent*, 1719–8429, 2016, https://www.ncbi.nlm.nih.gov/pmc/articles/PMC4879948/. Accessed 23 Nov. 2021.

50. Bear, Tracey L. K., et al. "The Role of the Gut Microbiota in Dietary Interventions for Depression and Anxiety." *OUP Academic*, Oxford University Press, 09 Mar. 2020, https://academic.oup.com/advances/article/11/4/890/5801053?login=true. Accessed 04 Feb. 2022.

51. Plaza-Díaz, Julio, et al. "Evidence of the Anti-Inflammatory Effects of Probiotics and Synbiotics in Intestinal Chronic Diseases." *Nutrients*, MDPI, 28 May 2017, https://www.ncbi.nlm.nih.gov/pmc/articles/PMC5490534/. Accessed 04 Feb. 2022.

52. Yaghoubfar, Rezvan, et al. "Modulation of Serotonin Signaling/Metabolism by *Akkermansia Muciniphila* and Its Extracellular Vesicles through the Gut-Brain Axis in Mice." Nature News, Nature Publishing Group, 17 Dec. 2020, https://www.nature.com/articles/s41598-020-79171-8. Accessed 04 Feb. 2022.

53. Starobrat-Hermelin, B., and T. Kozielec. "The Effects of Magnesium Physiological Supplementation on Hyperactivity in Children with Attention Deficit Hyperactivity Disorder (ADHD). Positive Response to Magnesium Oral Loading Test." *Magnesium Research*, U.S. National Library of Medicine, https://pubmed.ncbi.nlm.nih.gov/9368236/. Accessed 24 Nov. 2021.

54. Bilici, M., Yildirim, F., Kandil, S., Bekaroğlu, M., Yildirmiş, S., Değer, O., Ulgen, M., Yildiran, A., Aksu, H., "Double-Blind, Placebo-Controlled Study of Zinc Sulfate in the Treatment of Attention Deficit Hyperactivity Disorder." *Progress in Neuro-Psychopharmacology &*

Biological Psychiatry, U.S. National Library of Medicine, Jan. 2004, https://pubmed.ncbi.nlm.nih.gov/14687872/. Accessed 28 Jan. 2022.

55. Konofal, E., Lecendreux, M., Deron, J., Marchand, M., Cortese, S., Zaïm, M., Mouren, M. C., Arnulf, I., "Effects of Iron Supplementation on Attention Deficit Hyperactivity Disorder in Children." *Pediatric Neurology*, U.S. National Library of Medicine, Jan 2008, https://pubmed.ncbi.nlm.nih.gov/18054688/. Accessed 28 Jan. 2022.

56. Read more about *Rhodiola rosea* at this link: https://www.healthline.com/nutrition/rhodiola-rosea

57. Greenblatt, James. "Optimizing ADHD Treatment with Oligomeric Proanthocyanidins (OPCs)." *Psychiatry Redefined*, 20 Jan. *2018*, https://www.psychiatryredefined.org/optimizing-adhd-treatment-with-opcs/. Accessed 31 Jan. 2022.

58. ADDitude editors. "10 Foods (and Supplements and Vitamins!) to Boost Your ADHD Brain." *ADDitude*, ADDitude, Updated 05 Jan. 2022, https://www.additudemag.com/adhd-supplements-foods-vitamins/. Accessed 31 Jan. 2022.

59. Duke University Medical Center. "Zinc regulates communication between brain cells." *ScienceDaily*. ScienceDaily, 21 Sept. 2011. https://www.sciencedaily.com/releases/2011/09/110921132334.htm. Accessed 03 Feb. 2022.

60. Media, University of Toronto. "Zinc's Role in the Brain." *Media Room & Blue Book—University of Toronto*, 05 Oct. 2011, https://media.utoronto.ca/media-releases/health-medicine/zincs-role-in-the-brain/. Accessed 03 Feb. 2022.

61. Frye, Devon. "Children with ADHD Avoid Failure and Punishment More Than Others, Study Says." *ADDitude*, ADDitude, Updated 06 Nov. 2020, https://www.additudemag.com/children-with-adhd-avoid-failure-punishment/. Accessed 23 Dec. 2021.

62. White, Holly. "The Creativity of ADHD." *Scientific American*, Scientific American, 05 Mar. 2019, https://www.scientificamerican.com/article/the-creativity-of-adhd/. Accessed 02 Feb. 2022.

63. Flippin, Royce. "Hyperfocus: The ADHD Phenomenon of Intense Fixation." *ADDitude*, ADDitude, 03 Jan. 2022, https://www.additudemag.com/understanding-adhd-hyperfocus/. Accessed 02 Feb. 2022.

Made in United States
Orlando, FL
21 September 2024